The Salt Solution. DIET

Break Your Salt Addiction so You Can
Lose Weight,
Get Your Energy Back,
and **Live Longer!**

HEATHER K. JONES, RD,
WITH THE EDITORS OF **Prevention**® MAGAZINE

RODALE.

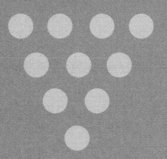

Contents

Introduction
Shake Out That Salt

S ALT. IT SEEMS HARMLESS ENOUGH. Sprinkle a dash here and there for an extra kick. But this flavor boost comes at a high price. Though salt (sodium chloride) often gets ignored by dieters and healthy eaters, it's actually one of the deadliest ingredients in the food supply. Yes, it's true!

Most of us have heard that a high sodium intake raises blood pressure, which in turn can cause heart attacks, strokes, and kidney disease. But did you know that overdoing it on salt has also been linked to dementia, diabetes, metabolic syndrome, osteoporosis, and cancer?[1, 2, 3] Some more salty news: High sodium can add inches to your waist. Yup, salt can make you fat.

Elevated levels of salt in the diet come from calorie-packed, nutrient-poor processed foods, such as those found in fast food and on many restaurant menus, as well as packaged food in supermarkets. As our lives have become increasingly more hectic and fast paced, salty processed and fast foods have become staples. That's not all. When you eat a lot of salt, it increases your thirst, especially for calorie-packed sodas. The bottom line: More salt equates to more calories, and this translates into higher numbers on the scale.

Unfortunately, most of us are seriously overdosing on sodium. The 2010 Dietary Guidelines for Americans, published by the Department of Health and Human Services and the Department of Agriculture, recommend that adults in general should consume no more than 2,300 milligrams (mg) of sodium per day—about 1 teaspoon. Persons who are 51 and older and those of any age who are African American or who have hypertension, diabetes, or chronic kidney disease should limit their daily sodium intake to only 1,500 milligrams. This was just revised from the previous recommendation of 2,300 milligrams because new research indicates that excess sodium is even more dangerous than previously thought. Instead, Americans on average consume 3,436 milligrams of sodium daily![4]

Slashing the salt in our diets can help our health, our waistlines, and even our wallets. One recent study found that if Americans reduced their salt intake by just ½ teaspoon a day, or 1,200 milligrams of sodium, the nation would save up to $24 billion a year in health care costs and the annual number of deaths would decrease by 44,000.[5] That's major savings on all fronts! (All this salt buzz has gotten officials talking about the best strategies to reduce salt in our food supply.) An Institute of Medicine report released in April 2010 recommends a new, coordinated approach to reduce sodium content in food gradually, one requiring new government standards for acceptable levels.[6] Meanwhile, New York City's health department has called on restaurant chains and food producers to lower the amount of salt in their products by 25 percent over the next 5 years.[7]

But you don't have to wait for regulations to kick in before taking charge of your health—and your waistline! That's why we've created the Salt Solution Diet. Over the next 6 weeks, this healthy eating program will lower your salt intake while helping you shed pounds and improve your overall health and increase your energy. The best part? This simple plan shows you how to slash salt consumption without having to change your entire diet or sacrifice flavor and taste. The Salt Solution is about what you can eat as opposed to what you should *not* eat. The more than 80 recipes in this book are not only delicious and satisfying, but also feature the Salt Solution Stars, powerful foods packed with the Miracle Minerals—potassium, magnesium, and calcium—that together work to counteract the negative effects of sodium on your body.[8]

Based on all the research we had unearthed linking sodium to obesity, hypertension, and many other health issues, we were confident that the Salt Solution would help people lose weight, lower their blood pressure, and improve their overall appearance, energy, and health. But of course a plan can deliver only if you follow it, so in order to make sure that our program is one that real men and women can fit into their busy lives, we asked 16 people to try it out. These dedicated men and women not only overcame their dangerous addiction to salt, they also lost pounds (up to almost 35 pounds in 6 weeks!) and inches (one woman lost 12¼ inches overall), increased energy, and gained confidence. Throughout this book you'll find words of encouragement in the inspiring stories of the men and women who participated in our panel and found their way back to eating the (low-salt and unprocessed) way nature intended.

The Salt Solution eating plan has two phases. It kicks off with the 2-Week Salt Solution Cleanse, designed to boost metabolism, increase energy, and banish bloat. Once you've purified your system and reset your taste buds, you'll start the 4-Week Shake the Salt Meal Plan. Both phases include lots of fruits and veggies, whole grains, lean protein, and filling fiber. The goal throughout the plan is to keep your sodium level at no more than 1,500 milligrams per day—the amount recommended to reduce chronic disease risk and maintain optimum health—while boosting your levels of the three Miracle Minerals.

The entire program is designed to cater to your tastes by allowing you to mix and match the recipes. Love a recipe? You can repeat it. You're also free to have a breakfast meal for dinner or even a lunch meal as a snack. Whatever works. Don't have time to cook every day? Learn smart strategies for eating out and choosing the best low-sodium (and minimally processed) packaged foods. This plan is really tailored for you, to fit your taste buds and needs.

Since eating well is only one component of living well, the Salt Solution also gives you tools to incorporate other healthy habits into your everyday life.

You'll learn how to reduce stress to help you conquer salty cravings. You'll find grocery shopping and cooking tips and tricks to help you create mouth-watering low-sodium meals on your own. If you're ready to get moving, try our 6-week Salt Solution Weight-Loss Workout. This easy fitness program will magnify all the benefits of the eating plan so that you lose even more weight, improve your energy and self-confidence, and combat disease!

Your healthy ways shouldn't end once the next 6 weeks are over. Remember, this plan isn't just a passing fad. It's a healthy eating and living plan for life. The Salt Solution Diet has been specially designed to allow you to maintain these habits for a lifetime, with your taste buds on board. So are you ready to start slashing that salt—and those pounds? Let's begin!

Understanding
SODIUM
OBESITY

Obesity rates in the United States are rising rapidly. Today almost 70 percent of American adults are overweight or obese, and it's become the single greatest threat to public health in this century.[1] Besides cutting calories and fat and increasing exercise, there's another important piece of the weight-loss puzzle: sodium intake. How can this nutrient, which is essential for health and contains no calories by itself, cause you to gain weight? Let's take a look at exactly what sodium is, where it's found, and the connection between sodium and obesity.

The Sodium Crisis

SOME SODIUM IS NECESSARY FOR HEALTH. This important mineral maintains the right balance of fluids in your body, helps transmit nerve impulses, and is important in muscle contraction and relaxation. Without sodium, you couldn't pick up your child, swim in a pool, or pull your hand away from a hot stove. Sodium is normally balanced with the help of your kidneys. If the sodium levels in your bloodstream are too low, your kidneys grab on to the

Sodium versus Salt

Although we're using "sodium" and "salt" interchangeably here, keep in mind that there is a difference. Table salt is actually sodium chloride (40 percent sodium and 60 percent chloride). And sodium is not only found in your salt-shaker, but also in foods and products that have been made with salt or one of its cousins, such as monosodium glutamate (MSG) and sodium bicarbonate (baking soda). Even some headache and heart-burn medicines contain sodium carbonate (two Alka-Seltzers, for example, have 1,134 milligrams). That's why sodium, not salt, is listed on nutrition labels.

Salt substitutes that are labeled "lite" or "low sodium" still contain sodium, just in lower amounts. These products often contain a mix of sodium chloride and potassium chloride. However, if products are labeled "sodium free," they are made only with potassium chloride and contain no sodium. Salt-free seasoning blends made with herbs and spices, including Mrs. Dash, are also sodium free.

The daily intake recommendations are given in milligrams of sodium. The table below explains how teaspoons of table salt translate to milligrams of sodium.

Salt to Sodium Equivalents

¹/₄ teaspoon salt	= 581 mg sodium
¹/₂ teaspoon salt	= 1,163 mg sodium
³/₄ teaspoon salt	= 1,744 mg sodium
1 teaspoon salt	= 2,325 mg sodium

salt that is present. When sodium levels are high, your kidneys excrete the excess in urine.

If you're healthy, don't worry about not getting enough sodium. You need only about 500 milligrams per day (that's slightly less than ¼ teaspoon of salt!) to keep your body working properly, and chances are, you're consuming five to seven times that, even if you never pick up a saltshaker. However, a variety of factors—including underlying medical conditions, severe vomiting and diarrhea, and, on rare occasions, excessive water intake during endurance activities—can cause sodium levels to drop, resulting in a condition known as *hyponatremia*. Symptoms include sluggishness, confusion, muscle twitching, and seizure. Hyponatremia can eventually lead to coma and death, but it's very rare in healthy adults. (It's most frequently seen in hospital and nursing home patients.) If you're healthy and eating a normal diet, you should have no problem getting the minimum amount of sodium you need.

The real problem lies in getting too much salt rather than too little. The issues start when we consume more sodium than our kidneys can handle. If the kidneys can't eliminate enough salt in urine, sodium starts to accumulate in blood. Sodium naturally attracts and holds water, which increases the total volume of the blood. This, in turn, makes your heart work harder to pump blood through your body, which increases your blood pressure. Not to mention that all that excess water in the blood will cause uncomfortable bloating and unsightly puffiness!

The average American eats far more than his recommended maximum of 1,500 milligrams of sodium per day. How much more? Data from 2005 to 2006 show that the average daily sodium intake for Americans over the age of 2 was almost 3,500 milligrams per day.[2]

In addition to causing high blood pressure, excess sodium intake may lead to stroke, coronary heart disease, cancer, kidney disease, dementia, diabetes, and bone loss. (We'll go into more detail on how salt can lead to all of these health problems in Chapter 2.) And, of course, there's sodium obesity. As our sodium intake continues to rise, so do obesity rates. Here's why.

The Scoop on Sodium Obesity

HAVE YOU EVER FELT FULL yet hungry at the same time? Or kept nibbling on snacks even after eating a big meal? One of the reasons salt is a favorite of chefs and food manufacturers alike is that salt enhances the inherent flavor of foods—that is, salt doesn't just make food taste salty, but it also makes sweet foods a little sweeter, sour foods a little tangier, and so on. In fact, the potato chip expression, "Betcha can't eat just one!" is true. Foods that scientists term "highly palatable," those with a high capacity to intensify appetite (like the hard-to-resist salty potato chips), alter brain chemistry in ways that promote overeating.

Brain scans show that consuming salt (as well as fat and sugar) causes the brain to release dopamine, the neurotransmitter associated with the pleasure center, making salty foods highly addictive—like nicotine and cocaine. In time, the brain gets hardwired, and this reward pathway can activate every time a person is reminded of a particular food (like when we see an advertisement), regardless of hunger. Couple this with the fact that we are surrounded by highly palatable (and inexpensive) salty and fatty processed foods—pretzels in the mall, pastries at the airport, doughnuts in the coffee shop, hot dogs at the ball game, French fries on the boardwalk, chips at service stations, and fast food, well, everywhere—and you create an environment ripe for overeating. Moreover, many salty foods—like French fries, potato chips, and fast-food sandwiches—are also high in fat and calories.

Hence, you have a salty catch-22. If you are eating a lot of salty foods, you're probably already consuming a relatively high number of calories, leading to weight gain. Eating salty foods makes you crave more salty foods, so you over-eat, leading to more weight gain. In addition, eating salty foods makes you thirsty. This wouldn't be an issue if you always turned to calorie-free and sodium-free plain water to slake your thirst. But that rarely proves to be the case. The increase in salt intake in the United States may help explain the simultaneous increase in the consumption of sugary beverages, which, in turn, has caused an increase in the intake of calories during the same period. Between 1977 and 2001, calorie intake from sweetened beverages increased by 135 percent in the United States. The net effect on energy intake was a 278-calorie increase per person per day. The American Heart Association has estimated that to burn off those 278 calories each American should now walk 1 hour 10 minutes more every day than they did in 1977.

The Science of Table Salt

Table salt is sodium chloride, a chemical combination made from one atom of sodium and one of chlorine. Separately, sodium is an extremely volatile metal and chlorine is a gas, but together they form the harmless white grains you sprinkle on popcorn. You've probably heard of iodized salt. That's table salt with a small amount of iodine added. This practice started to prevent iodine deficiency, a serious condition that can lead to goiter (swelling of the thyroid gland) and mental retardation. We need a small amount of iodine per day, but it's not found in too many foods. Kelp is an excellent source of iodine; and yogurt, milk, eggs, and strawberries are all very good sources. Even with these food sources, many populations are susceptible to iodine deficiency. In the 1920s, scientists in the United States started pressing the salt industry to add iodine to table salt. Now, most commercially available table salt contains iodine.

Sure, you expect potato chips to be high in salt, but lots of foods naturally contain sodium. You can get all the sodium you need from these healthy, whole foods. The problem is sodium lurking in processed foods.

BEETS = 64 milligrams sodium (per 1 medium beet)

CELERY = 96 milligrams sodium (per 3 ribs)

1% MILK = 107 milligrams (per 1 cup)

ARTICHOKES = 120 milligrams sodium (per 1 medium artichoke)

SHRIMP = 126 milligrams sodium (per 3 ounces)

KELLOGG'S RAISIN BRAN CEREAL = 350 milligrams sodium (per 1 cup)

KRAFT LIGHT N' LIVELY COTTAGE CHEESE = 420 milligrams sodium (per 1/2 cup)

CLASSICO TOMATO AND BASIL PASTA SAUCE = 470 milligrams sodium (per 1/2 cup)

PILLSBURY GRANDS! HOME-STYLE BISCUITS = 600 milligrams sodium (per biscuit)

GREEN GIANT REGULAR CUT GREEN BEANS = 800 milligrams sodium (per 1 cup)

DELI TURKEY MEAT = 900 milligrams sodium (per 75 grams)

Regrettably, this has not happened. Only 3 in 10 American adults get the recommended amount of physical activity and 37 percent report that they are not physically active at all.[3] In 2 decades—from 1976 to 2002—the prevalence of obesity was 120 percent higher among men and 99 percent higher among women.[4] In addition, these trends paralleled the rising obesity seen in this country.[5] One study found that if the amount of sodium in a child's diet was cut in half, their consumption of sugary beverages would decrease by about 2 per week.[6] In adults, cutting sodium in half would reduce fluid intake by about 350 milliliters per day.[7] Since studies have shown that a good portion of fluid intake comes from sugary, caloric beverages, a reduction in total fluid intake by cutting salt could cut calories and help people lose weight.

Eating too much salt may also cause obesity in less noticeable ways than increased thirst or hunger. Studies in animals have shown that a high-salt diet increased the size of fat cells.[8] Animal studies have also shown that a high salt intake increased the insulin levels in blood.[9] Insulin is a hormone that determines whether we burn fat or store it. After you eat a meal, the sugars (glucose) in your blood are absorbed and then transported to the liver, where they are stored as glycogen. When you need energy, this glycogen is broken down and converted to glucose to fuel your body. However, when the capacity of your liver to store glycogen is reached, insulin causes the excess glucose to be converted into fatty acids, which are then transported to adipose, or fat, tissue. In other words, insulin tells your body to store sugars in the blood as fat—so the more salt you eat, the more insulin you may have; the more insulin you have, the more fat you store and the more weight you gain.

There may also be an evolutionary aspect to our high sodium intakes. Because we need sodium for bodily functions, our bodies may be hardwired to appreciate and search out salty flavors.[10] Our early hunter-gatherer ancestors ate mostly vegetarian diets that were naturally low in sodium, and so their bodies evolved to conserve sodium. The addition of large quantities of sodium to our diets is a relatively recent innovation (see Salty Times on page 14), and our bodies cannot handle the increased load. Salt was once so valuable that it influenced trade routes, provoked wars, and was used as medicine to treat a wide variety of ailments. However, in our society, salt is anything but scarce, so this preference for high-sodium foods is doing us a lot more harm than good.

Another important reason to lower sodium is to achieve nutritional balance. As we noted earlier, the foods in our diet that supply the most salt tend to be loaded not just with sodium but also with calories, saturated fat, and cholesterol. This type of salty, fatty, and processed fare crowds out more healthful options that will fill you up, keep you energized, and set you up for weight-loss success. Salt Solution fare, on the other hand, includes delicious and satisfying whole foods, such as fruits, veggies, whole grains, and lean meat.

Finally, as many of us have learned from personal experience, eating lots of salty foods can cause bloating. Sodium in your bloodstream causes you to retain water, in some cases adding as much as a pound or two and causing you to feel sluggish, puffy, and uncomfortable. Sure, the water weight packed on from eating too much sodium is temporary (unlike the weight from excess calories, which is stored as fat), but it's still a problem. When your favorite pair of jeans won't button, it doesn't matter where that extra pudge is coming from. Cutting out the salt helps you drop the water weight almost immediately.

Processed, Packaged, and Prepared, Oh My!

Convenience food is commercially produced for ease of consumption; and processed, packaged, and prepared foods all fall under this umbrella term. We use these words pretty much interchangeably to describe the sodium-packed foods you should avoid. However, there are some slight differences, and not all these foods are bad for your health.

PROCESSED describes any food that has been changed from its natural, raw state by canning, freezing, dehydrating, or pasteurizing. Processing can result in healthy food choices—like freezing fresh vegetables or pasteurizing fat-free milk. But processing can also result in high-sodium foods, like super-salty canned soups and deli meats.

PACKAGED simply means that a food has been packed for transportation and sale, such as bagged spinach or cartons of berries. This can describe fresh, natural, whole foods. However, preservatives are frequently added to packaged foods to protect them from spoiling during shipping.

PREPARED foods are items you can buy that are ready to eat. Think anything from a restaurant or supermarket take-out section. Since most prepared foods aren't required to have nutrition labels, often you have no idea how much sodium they contain. A better idea: Use the easy recipes in this book to make your own delicious low-salt meals.

The Sodium Supply

MAYBE YOU'RE THINKING, I'll just lay off the saltshaker. The problem is that the vast majority of the salt we consume is hidden in processed, packaged, and prepared foods. In fact, about 80 percent of the sodium we eat is found in the premade crackers, cookies, cereals, soups, frozen dinners, and pasta sauces in the grocery aisles or in foods eaten outside the home.[11] Why exactly do food manufacturers need so much sodium? Here's a rundown of the most common uses of salt in food processing.

Preservative: Salt dehydrates bacteria in foods, inhibiting bacterial growth and food spoilage. Manufacturers add salt so their products can stay on shelves longer.

Texture: Salt helps add consistency to foods' textures. It's used in breads and other grain products to strengthen and smooth the dough. In cured meats like salami and ham, salt improves tenderness by allowing the meat proteins to bind more water. Salt also promotes consistency in the texture of cheeses.

Binding: Salt helps mixtures of meats (like sausages and deli meats) bind and emulsify together.

Fermentation control: Fermentation is necessary to produce breads and other baked products, pickles, cheese, and sauerkraut. Salt controls the speed of fermentation to produce uniform products.

Color development: Salt is often combined with compounds called nitrates in processed meats like hot dogs to produce color. Salt also helps bread crust to brown during baking.

Food safety: Salt is required in the production of smoked fish and cured meats to control bacteria and microbes.

(continued on page 13)

9

WHAT'S YOUR
SALT-O-METER SCORE?

Since so many sources of sodium are hidden, it can be hard to tell if you're getting too much. Take this quiz to determine your Salt-o-Meter. Choose all of the answers that apply to you.

1. WHEN I NEED A TREAT, I REACH FOR:

A. A piece of dark chocolate

B. French fries from my favorite fast-food restaurant

C. A cookie from a coffee shop

D. A piece of fresh fruit

Answers: *Give yourself 1 point for choice B or C. You probably guessed that French fries are salty even if you don't add any salt to them, but did you know that a ginger molasses cookie from Starbucks contains 340 milligrams of sodium? If you have a sweet tooth, try a piece of dark chocolate; 1 ounce contains 150 calories, 30 milligrams of sodium, and healthy antioxidants. Fresh fruit is your best choice.*

2. I ALWAYS TOP MY BURGERS WITH:

A. Ketchup and mustard

B. A slice of cheese

C. Lettuce and tomato

D. Pickles

Answers: *Give yourself 1 point for choice A, B, or D. Ketchup, mustard, regular cheese, and pickles are all very high-sodium burger toppings— about 200 milligrams per serving for ketchup, 50 milligrams per serving for mustard, 350 milligrams per serving for cheese, and 200 milligrams per serving for pickles.*

3. TO QUENCH MY THIRST, I DRINK:

A. Gatorade

B. Water

C. Diet soda

D. Regular soda

Answers: *Give yourself 1 point for choice A. Gatorade contains salt to replace sodium lost through sweating. Unless you're an endurance athlete, skip the Gatorade. And while regular soda is low in sodium, it contains tons of calories. Your best bet: water.*

4. WHEN I HAVE AN UPSET STOMACH, I TAKE:

A. Pepto-Bismol

B. An antacid like Alka-Seltzer

C. Nothing, I wait it out

D. Chamomile tea

Answers: *Give yourself 1 point for choice B. Alka-Seltzer contains sodium bicarbonate. Taking it once in a while is fine, but you can also ask your doctor for sodium-free alternatives.*

5. AT THE BAR, I CHOOSE A:

A. Vodka tonic

B. Beer

C. Glass of wine

D. Bloody Mary

Answers: *Give yourself 1 point for choice D. Vodka contains no sodium and beer and wine very little. But the tomato juice in a Bloody Mary is salt-packed—about 650 milligrams of sodium per cup of tomato juice! And Bloody Marys are often served with high-sodium garnishes like pickles.*

6. **FOR BREAKFAST, I NORMALLY EAT:**

A. A multigrain bagel and cream cheese

B. Raisin bran cereal with fat-free milk

C. A Lärabar and a latte

D. Pancakes

Answers: *Give yourself 1 point for choices A, B, and D. A bagel can contain more than 600 milligrams of sodium, and raisin bran cereal can have more than 250 milligrams of sodium per serving. Pancakes from McDonald's have 590 milligrams of sodium (not including butter or syrup!), but if you think making pancakes at home is best, be careful—many mixes contain more than 700 milligrams of sodium per serving.*

7. **TO SPICE UP MY CHILI, I ADD:**

A. Salsa I buy from the supermarket

B. Salsa I make myself

C. Tabasco sauce

D. A shake of cayenne pepper

Answers: *Give yourself 1 point for choice A. Commercially prepared*

salsa is usually high in sodium. Make it yourself, and you can use only fresh vegetables (and maybe a tiny sprinkle of salt). The original flavor of Tabasco sauce has about 2 milligrams of sodium per serving, and pure cayenne pepper is salt free.*

8. **FOR LUNCH, I NORMALLY EAT:**

A. Sandwich on whole wheat bread with deli turkey and a slice of cheese

B. Canned soup

C. Caesar salad with grilled chicken

D. Sushi with soy sauce and pickled ginger

Answers: *Unfortunately, you'll need to give yourself 1 point for each of these answers. All these foods have very high-sodium ingredients—deli turkey, canned soup, Caesar salad dressing, and soy sauce and pickled ginger. The good news is that you can make small substitutions to lower the sodium: Choose low-sodium deli meats and cheeses, low-sodium canned soup, make your own salad with salt-free grilled chicken and homemade dressing, and skip the soy sauce and pickled ginger with your sushi.*

(Continued)

WHAT'S YOUR
SALT-O-METER SCORE? *(CONTINUED)*

9. **ON MY SALADS, I USE:**

   A. Oil and vinegar

   B. Bottled regular salad dressing

   C. Bottled low-fat or fat-free salad
   dressing

   D. Croutons

   Answers: *Give yourself 1 point for
   choices B, C, and D. Bottled dressings and prepared croutons are very
   high in sodium. Instead, make your
   own dressing with a drizzle of olive oil
   and your favorite vinegar. For crunch,
   top your salads with a few unsalted
   nuts instead of croutons.*

10. **MY FAVORITE FROZEN
    DESSERT IS:**

    A. A chocolate malted milk shake

    B. An ice cream sundae with the works

    C. A dish of soft-serve

    D. Fruit sorbet

    Answers: *Give yourself 1 point for
    choices A and B. Malt powder is high
    in sodium, and an ice cream sundae
    may contain high-sodium ingredients
    like salted nuts.*

**ADD UP YOUR POINTS TO CALCULATE
YOUR PERSONAL SALTOMETER.**

0–5. **LOW**
Congratulations! You're
doing well watching your sodium intake.
Use the Salt Solution plan to help you
reinforce the good work you're doing and
for tips to reduce your sodium intake
even more.

6–10. **MEDIUM**
You're moving in the right
direction. Use the Salt Solution plan to
help you remove those last few salt
sources. Once you banish them from your
diet, you'll improve your health—and your
waistline—even more.

11–15: **HIGH**
You're approaching
dangerous levels! Start the Salt Solution
plan to get your sodium intake back into
the safe zone. If you don't act soon, your
health could be permanently affected.

16–21: **DANGER**
You need to put the Salt
Solution rules into effect ASAP. You're
probably already feeling the effects of a
high-sodium lifestyle, including bloating,
and you may already have high blood
pressure. Use the Salt Solution plan to
start moving your numbers down.

Of course, you can't stop eating out, and we don't expect you to give up the convenience of packaged foods entirely. In Chapter 7, we'll give you all the tips and tools you need to shop smart and identify which products are really low in sodium (and still taste good!). In Chapter 8, you'll learn how to read a menu for hidden sources of sodium.

The remaining 20 percent of salt we consume is what we add at the table or in cooking or what naturally occurs in food. There are also many high-sodium condiments (mustard, soy sauce) and ingredients (pickles, olives) that add sodium to your daily tally. And then there's the sodium that's found naturally in some foods. Celery, milk, meat, and shellfish, among many other foods, contain sodium. Should you cut these foods from your diet? Of course not. Just be aware that even when you eat an all-natural diet with no added salt, you'll still consume some sodium—which is necessary for your body to function properly.

Prescription and over-the-counter drugs are two final sources of sodium that you should be aware of. Some antacids, laxatives, and nonsteroidal

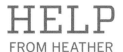

HELP
FROM HEATHER

How can I tell if I'm sensitive to salt?

Salt-sensitive individuals are people who are more sensitive to the effects of sodium. These people retain sodium more easily, which leads to fluid retention and increased blood pressure with lower salt intakes. So how do you know if you're salt sensitive?

Some Americans are more likely than others to be salt sensitive, including older people, African Americans, people with salt-sensitive family members, or people with a parent, sibling, or child with hypertension. (Researchers have estimated that about a quarter of Americans with normal blood pressure levels and about 58 percent of those with hypertension are salt sensitive.[12]) The problem is that there's no reliable predictor or test of salt sensitivity. The bottom line: Everyone should live a low-sodium lifestyle.

anti-inflammatory drugs (NSAIDs) contain considerable amounts of sodium. The Food and Drug Administration issued rules requiring labeling for over-the-counter drugs that contain levels of sodium that may be harmful for people with certain conditions. Ask your physician about the sodium content of the medications you're taking.

Salty Times

S
O NOW YOU KNOW that almost 80 percent of the salt we consume comes from processed and prepared foods. But how did our food supply become so salty?

Since ancient times, salt has been used as a flavor enhancer and as a preservative. As we described earlier, salt improves the taste and texture of

A Salt by Any Other Name ...

BLACK SALT, also known as kala namak, is a condiment used in India. It's actually pink or purple, not black. Black salt is made primarily of sodium chloride with a small percentage of sulfur and other minerals.

FLEUR DE SEL is a type of sea salt that's hand harvested off the coast of France.

KOSHER SALT was developed for the preparation of kosher meats. It contains coarser grains than table salt and is iodine free.

ROCK SALT is nonfood-grade salt used to melt ice on sidewalks and roads in the winter.

SEA SALT is unrefined salt that's collected by evaporating seawater. Sea salt is 98 percent sodium chloride; the rest is made up of minerals like iron, sulfur, and magnesium. Sea salt is often more flavorful than table salt as a result of this mineral component.

many foods. Salt kills bacteria that might cause spoiling and also draws the moisture out of food, thus preventing more bacteria from growing. Before refrigeration, salt was used to preserve fish and meat for later consumption. Hunters would kill a large animal, and meat that wasn't eaten immediately was salted so it didn't spoil. The demand for salt led to the development of early trade routes throughout Europe and Asia, and industrialization accelerated salt's popularity.

Salt became cheap and widely available, and it quickly developed into one of the first mass-market food additives. Because salt masks flavors produced in processing (like metallic and chemical aftertastes), it helps food taste more savory and sweet (by making it easier for our taste receptors to recognize sweetness) and provides an almost addictive taste combination with fat and sugar to keep customers snacking, it is added to a plethora of commercially produced foods.

Cutting salt from processed foods would require companies to use more expensive fresh ingredients—like pricey, but tastier, fresh herbs in canned soups instead of cheaper, blander, dried herbs. With all the focus on low-fat and low-calorie foods, adding salt is an easy way to increase flavor without increasing fat or calories. But as you'll learn from this book, this extra sodium can also cause weight gain, just like too many grams of fat or calories.

Industry insiders say that cutting salt doesn't have the same market potential for profit that cutting calories or fat has. According to Dr. Howard Moskowitz, a food scientist and consultant to major food manufacturers, "If all of a sudden people would demand lower salt because low salt makes them look younger, this [oversalted food supply] problem would be solved overnight."

Cutting salt from your diet will in fact make you look and feel younger since it reduces bloating, helps you lose weight, and improves your overall health. A recent study looked at the preventable causes of death in the United

States, including high cholesterol, high blood pressure, physical inactivity, and poor dietary habits.[13] Among the dietary factors studied, a high-salt diet was shown to have the largest effect on preventable deaths, accounting for 4 percent of deaths in American adults. Because of research like this, over the past few years, pressure has been mounting on the food industry to reduce the amount of salt in products. Research has shown that voluntary reduction of sodium by the food industry could cut Americans' salt intake by 9.5 percent (a small reduction that you would not notice), which could extend the lives of Americans by 1.3 million years collectively. This reduction would also save $32.1 billion in health care costs.[14] The food industry is currently researching ways to decrease sodium content without sacrificing taste, including changing the shape of salt crystals so they feel different in the mouth. But significant cuts in the sodium content of food are still a long way off. Researching and developing new products is expensive and consumers aren't yet demanding low-sodium foods in the same way they're demanding low-fat and low-calorie foods.

We can't wait around for the food industry to change their products (though we certainly should demand that they do!). A better, immediate way to decrease your salt intake? Cut back on the amount of processed and prepared foods you eat and live the Salt Solution way!

The Salt Solution Strategy

HOW ARE YOU GOING TO CUT SALT from your diet and lose weight? Easy—on the Salt Solution Diet, you'll limit your sodium intake to no more than 1,500 milligrams per day—the amount recommended to reduce the risk of chronic disease—while you increase potassium, calcium, and magnesium. These three Miracle Minerals counteract the negative effects of excess sodium, and upping their intake (while decreasing sodium) will bring your body into balance and (bonus!) reduce bloating. You'll be eating a lot fewer processed and chemically enhanced foods on this plan, which will cleanse your palate and set you up for a lifetime of low-salt living. We'll even teach you how to grocery shop and eat out the Salt Solution way. You'll not only drop pounds, you'll break your unhealthy salt addiction. The low-salt tips and tricks you'll learn in this book will teach you how to make these healthy changes stick!

We'll teach you how to handle emotional and mindless eating. Have you found yourself eating not because of hunger, but because of boredom, stress, or sadness? This is emotional eating. Mindless eating is the eating you do automatically, without even noticing, like consuming an entire bag of potato chips in front of the television. The Salt Solution will teach you techniques to deal with emotional and mindless eating, like how to tell the difference between physical and emotional hunger and how keeping a journal can help you recognize what emotions cause you to reach for the cookies. Not only will these techniques teach you more about yourself, they'll also help you cut unnecessary calories and sodium from your diet. You'll also learn the Salt Solution techniques to keep a positive attitude in case you hit a roadblock. We know that, like any major change in life, losing weight and improving your health by slashing sodium will come with difficulties, but you'll have the skills to deal with any unexpected challenges.

The Salt Solution also includes a 6-week exercise plan designed by a fitness expert, so you can lose weight and feel better faster. You won't need expensive equipment, a gym membership, or tons of free time, either. Our exercise plan is designed to be fun, flexible, and easy to follow; and it can be customized to your fitness level. If any exercise is too difficult for you, try the Make It Easier option; if any exercise is way too easy, you can opt to do the Make It Harder option instead.

Finally, the Salt Solution will provide you with more than 80 delicious recipes. Not a cook? Don't worry; these recipes are easy to prepare and will give you confidence in the kitchen. If you want suggestions for when you're in a hurry, we list the best ready-made meals and bars that you can grab and go. We'll also teach you the building blocks of healthy meals so you can be your own dietitian and create your own healthy, low-salt meals.

First, you'll start with the 2-Week Salt Solution Cleanse to boost your metabolism, increase your energy, and cleanse your system of sodium, saturated fat, and trans fat; you'll reset your taste buds. The cells in our taste buds turn over every 1 to 2 weeks, so by the end of the 2-Week Cleanse, your taste buds will rejuvenate and you'll begin to savor the subtle flavors in real foods.

Once you've detoxed, you'll start the 4-Week Shake the Salt Meal Plan, which will include four delicious, healthy, low-salt meals a day plus a Mineral Boost Juice. You'll slash salt consumption without having to change your entire diet and without sacrificing flavor and taste. You'll feel great and look even better.

After 6 weeks of the Salt Solution, you'll be feeling leaner, less bloated, and more energetic. Also, you'll probably notice a difference on the scale and perhaps in your blood pressure reading. Are you finished? Definitely not! The Salt Solution is a program you can follow to reach your final weight-loss and health goals and to stay there for the rest of your life. We'll provide you with the techniques you need to stay low salt for life.

The Salt Solution Breakdown

The 2-Week Salt Solution Cleanse

In just 2 weeks you can rev up your metabolism, increase your energy, and cleanse your system of excess sodium, bad fats, and other harmful substances. You will reset your taste buds, too, an important part of the Salt Solution strategy. The Cleanse includes:

- **Three satisfying 300-calorie meals** per day, each featuring a Salt Solution Star, designed to jump-start weight loss and eliminate bloating caused by salt.
- **A daily Mineral Boost Juice**, a smoothie pumped with the Miracle Minerals and other nutrients you need to get your body back into balance. Choose from three delicious varieties.

The 4-Week Shake the Salt Meal Plan

At the end of this program, you'll be leaner and on your way to a healthier, low-salt lifestyle! You'll enjoy 4 weeks of delicious nutrient-packed meals and recipes you can mix and match. The plan consists of:

- **Four filling 300-calorie meals** per day. Choose from the quick-fix Cleanse meals or from the more than 80 Salt Solution recipes.
- **A daily dose of Mineral Boost Juice**. This tasty concoction, available in three flavors, keeps your health at an optimum level while you drop pounds.

An Optional Exercise Program

You already have the best weight-loss equipment—your feet. The secret is knowing how to use them. The optional Salt Solution Weight-Loss Workout includes a walking program designed to turn your body into a more efficient calorie- and fat-burning machine. The Salt Solution strength-training routine will help you develop even more muscle so you can burn even more calories.

Salt Solution Success Story

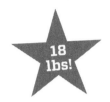

18 lbs!

Shannon Ferry

Age: 35

Pounds Lost: 18

Inches Lost: 11½ overall

SHANNON FERRY, A 35-YEAR-OLD TEACHER, used to be able to eat whatever she wanted. As a collegiate volleyball player, she followed a vigorous exercise regimen, but when her volleyball career ended, the weight gain started. "When I was not as active as I used to be and not required to work out, my weight gain began. I was so used to being able to eat and drink whatever I wanted without weight gain, that I continued those habits."

Shannon did what many people do—she promised herself she'd start her diet *tomorrow*. Whenever she got too unhappy with her weight, she turned to different diet programs. On these programs, she lost weight but then always went back to her old habits. Shannon found that she succeeded with the Salt Solution for one simple reason: "The Salt Solution isn't a diet, it's a lifestyle change. It's not about cutting out all carbs or cutting out all fat, it's about recognizing the nutrients that are most beneficial to your body and recognizing the foods and additives that are harmful." Shannon was surprised by the Salt Solution meals. "I was always double-checking the amounts because it always seemed like there was too much food! I'm amazed with how much I can eat and how satisfied I feel when I'm eating fresh whole foods."

The Salt Solution has cured Shannon of her salt addiction. "Since I started this plan, my salt cravings became nonexistent. I don't need salty foods anymore. I love that I can now taste subtle flavors instead of just saltiness in my food." Has Shannon's energy increased? "YES! Since being on this plan, I've started waking up more refreshed, and I find that I am more energized throughout the day. And I never need a 3:00 p.m. sugary snack anymore, which used to be a daily habit."

SALT SOLUTION MAKEOVER

Shannon's "**Before**" Diet

- **BREAKFAST:** 3 cups Golden Grahams cereal, 2 cups 1% milk, 1 cup orange juice
- **LUNCH:** 2 slices of plain pizza, cup of blueberry yogurt, 2 string cheeses
- **SNACK:** Snickers bar
- **DINNER:** Baked seasoned chicken breast, boiled green beans, Rice-a-Roni rice
- **DESSERT:** Slice of cheesecake

Shannon's "**After**" Diet

- **BREAKFAST:** Banana-Spinach Smoothie
- **LUNCH:** Mini Pizza, spinach salad, 2 small clementines
- **SNACK:** Cranberries-on-a-Banana
- **DINNER:** Penne Bolognese with a large mixed vegetable salad

"**Before**" Nutrition

- **Calories:** 3,218
- **Sodium:** 5,649 mg
- **Saturated Fat:** 42.4 g
- **Fiber:** 18 g

"**After**" Nutrition

- **Calories:** 1,454
- **Sodium:** 676 mg
- **Saturated Fat:** 10 g
- **Fiber:** 28 g

Salt Solution Improvements: Before starting the Salt Solution, Shannon's diet was chockful of salty items like pizza and Rice-a-Roni. Shannon tends to eat four times a day (instead of the typical Salt Solution five) and is filling up on her very own Salt Solution creations. She has slashed her caloric and sodium intakes (3,218 calories to 1,454 calories and 5,649 mg sodium to 676 mg sodium), and she looks and feels wonderful. On the Salt Solution, Shannon not only lost 18 pounds and an amazing 11½", but her blood pressure dropped from 130/80 mmHg to 120/66 mmHg.

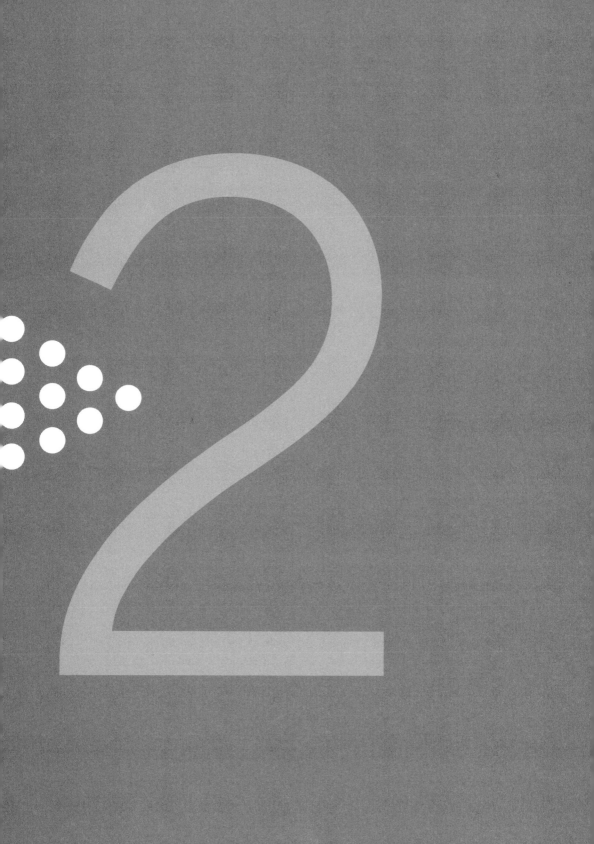

SODIUM, THE SILENT KILLER

Most people put sodium low on their list of worries, assuming it's not that big a deal unless their blood pressure starts to climb. High blood pressure, or hypertension, *is* a problem; it increases your risk of dying of a heart attack or stroke more than any other risk factor, including smoking and high cholesterol. However, high blood pressure is just the tip of the iceberg. The truth is that everyone needs to be concerned about sodium. Salt may harm your brain, kidneys, and other organs beyond its effect on blood pressure.

So just how bad are the effects of too much salt in your diet? You already know that sodium is a major foe in the battle of the bulge—and of course being overweight is itself a risk factor for many health conditions, but did you know that the evidence linking salt to a host of serious health issues is mounting? Let's examine the research.

Know Your Numbers

Why is it important to get your blood pressure checked? Most people with hypertension have no symptoms, even if they have high blood pressure. (If your blood pressure is extremely high, you may experience symptoms like severe headache, vision problems, chest pain, difficulty breathing, or irregular heartbeat.) Without getting regular blood pressure readings, you may not know your blood pressure is high until it's too late and you've already suffered the health effects. You should get your blood pressure checked by a physician at least every 2 years after age 20, and you may need more frequent readings if you have already been diagnosed with hypertension or prehypertension or if you have other cardiovascular disease risk factors.

Blood pressure measurements are taken in millimeters of mercury (mmHg) and are given as two numbers. The first is your systolic blood pressure (the pressure created when your heart beats) and the second is your diastolic blood pressure (the pressure inside blood vessels when your heart is resting). The following chart reflects blood pressure categories defined by the American Heart Association.

Blood Pressure Category	Systolic mmHg (Upper #)		Diastolic mmHg (Lower #)
Normal	Less than 120	and	Less than 80
Prehypertension high blood pressure	120–139	or	80–89
(Hypertension) Stage 1 high blood pressure	140–159	or	90–99
(Hypertension) Stage 2	160 or higher	or	100 or higher
Hypertensive crisis (emergency care needed)	Higher than 180	or	Higher than 110

Source: American Heart Association

High Blood Pressure

W E KNOW INCREASED SODIUM INTAKE raises blood pressure, which, in turn, increases your risk of heart disease and stroke. Worldwide, high blood pressure is the biggest cause of death and the second-biggest cause of disability. In fact, increased blood pressure is the largest contributor to stroke and coronary heart disease, accounting for 62 percent of strokes and 49 percent of coronary heart disease.[1] Hypertension increases your risk of dying of a heart attack or stroke more than any other risk factor—including smoking, high cholesterol, and obesity. In addition, it harms your kidneys, brain, sleep patterns, and even your sex life.

One of every three Americans has hypertension, another one of three has prehypertension. Among people with hypertension, it's not well managed: 65 percent of Americans who have hypertension don't have it under control, or

HELP
FROM HEATHER

Should you take drugs for hypertension?

If your blood pressure is between 120/80 mmHg and 139/89 mmHg, your doctor will likely recommend lifestyle changes before prescribing medication. These include following a healthy, low-sodium diet (like the Salt Solution), not smoking, maintaining a healthy weight, exercising at least 30 minutes most days of the week, and limiting the amount of alcohol you drink (no more than 1 drink a day for women and 2 a day for men).

If your blood pressure is over 140/90 mmHg, your doctor may prescribe antihypertensive medication. But remember, even if you're on medication, you should still follow the healthy lifestyle habits listed above in order to get off the medication!

There are dozens of medications for hypertension out there. Whether you need to take drugs for your high blood pressure is up to you and your physician.

below 140/90 millimeters of mercury (mmHg).[2] And unfortunately, the probability that you will have normal blood pressure your whole life is unlikely. At some point in their lifetimes, 90 percent of all Americans will develop hypertension.[3] Currently, more than 25 percent of the world's population has high blood pressure.[4]

Much of this is a result of sodium intake. Sodium intake is directly related to blood pressure levels in adults and children. When you eat too much salt, your kidneys (the body's natural filter) can't excrete the excess and the surplus salt stays in your bloodstream. Increased salt in the blood attracts water (and causes bloating), which increases your total blood volume and makes the heart work harder to pump blood through your body. Voilà! Increased blood pressure. New research also shows that salt raises blood pressure because it makes it harder for the cardiovascular system (your heart, blood, and blood vessels) to juggle the regulation of blood pressure and body temperature at the same time.[5] With increased salt consumption comes increased blood pressure. It's just that simple. Inversely, less salt means lower blood pressure. Multiple studies in adults and children have shown that cutting salt lowers blood pressure.[6, 7] And a recent analysis of 13 studies found that people who decreased their salt intake not only lowered their blood pressure but also their risk of heart attacks and strokes.[8]

Atherosclerosis and Aneurysms

NORMAL, HEALTHY ARTERIES ARE SMOOTH so blood can flow freely through them. Excess sodium consumption, as we know, causes high blood pressure, which damages arterial cells, making the artery walls thick and stiff, a process called *arteriosclerosis*.[9] This progresses into atherosclerosis, a condition in which fats from your diet enter your bloodstream and stick to the damaged artery cells and walls. Enough fat cells stuck to your artery walls can cause a blockage of blood. Australian researchers put people with normal blood pressure on typical (approximately 3,500 milligrams of sodium per day) or low-salt (about 1,150 milligrams of sodium per day) diets for 2 weeks. Study subjects who ate the typical-salt diet had stiffer arteries (and higher blood pressure) than people who ate the low-salt diets.[10]

This doesn't just happen in your heart's arteries; it can also affect your brain, kidneys, arms, and legs. Atherosclerosis can lead to a number of serious problems, including chest pain, heart attack, heart failure, kidney failure, stroke, peripheral arterial disease, and aneurysm.

An *aneurysm* is a bulge in the wall of an artery that can occur anywhere in your body—kidneys, heart, brain, arms, and legs. Aneurysms are caused by weakening of the blood vessels from high blood pressure. When they rupture, they cause massive internal bleeding and can be life-threatening.

Heart Disease

ALTHOUGH HEART DISEASE is no longer the automatic death sentence it once was, it remains a leading killer of both men and women. Heart disease is the number one killer in the United States and is responsible for 40 percent of all deaths.[11] If you have been diagnosed with any type of heart disease (or have risk factors for heart disease), you've most likely already been advised to cut back on sodium in your diet. Doctors have long known that a low-salt diet can help guard against heart disease.

Your prognosis is worse if you have high blood pressure, which of course is a likely result of a high-sodium diet. People with hypertension are more likely to die of a heart attack than people who don't have high blood pressure. High blood pressure damages your heart by making it work harder to pump blood. The heart is a muscle, and just like other muscles in your body that enlarge when you work them harder, your heart enlarges with more work. But building muscle in your heart is not a good thing. An enlarged heart muscle (also known as *left ventricular hypertrophy*) increases your risk of heart failure, heart attack, and sudden death. Over time, your heart will weaken from the strain of pumping blood at high pressure. Heart failure will eventually occur when your heart simply can't work any longer.[12]

A high salt intake has also been shown to cause *myocardial fibrosis,* the formation of scar tissue, which suggests that excessive salt consumption may be an important factor in the development of cardiovascular disease.[13] Fibrosis can lead to heart disease by limiting the extent that the heart muscle can expand, which leads to irregularities in blood pressure and ultimately heart failure. Other studies show that consuming too much sodium may increase arterial pressure in the left ventricle (the chamber on the left side of the heart). These data suggest that sodium itself, not the high blood pressure caused by sodium, may be dangerous to your heart.[14, 15]

The good news is that just a small change in your salt intake can make a big difference in your risk of heart disease. Researchers at the Federico II University of Naples found that a decrease of just 5 grams of sodium per day was associated with as much as a 17 percent lower risk of heart disease.[16] In the Trials of Hypertension Prevention, 2,400 people with prehypertension were either assigned a lower-salt diet (1,800 milligrams of sodium per day) or told to follow more general guidelines for healthy eating (including information about how to lose weight). Ten to 15 years after the study ended, the researchers went back to look at the study participants. The people in the lower-salt group had a 25 to 30 percent lower risk of heart attacks, strokes, or other cardiovascular problems as well as a 20 percent lower risk of death from cardiovascular disease compared to the people in the general healthy eating group.[17]

Kidney Disease

KIDNEYS ARE YOUR BODY'S FILTERS; they remove impurities and excess fluid from your blood for excretion. They also balance the amount of sodium stored in your body for optimal health. When your sodium levels are low, your kidneys hold on to the sodium; when levels are high, they excrete the excess in urine.

Over time, though, if you continue to eat too much salt and sodium levels stay high, you will develop hypertension, which will make your heart work harder and eventually can damage blood vessels throughout your body, including the kidneys. If these specialized blood vessels, called *glomeruli*, are damaged from high blood pressure, they can't work.[18] This leads to kidney disease, kidney failure, scarring, and kidney artery aneurysm.

Scarring to the kidneys is known as *renal fibrosis*, and it's the main cause of kidney failure requiring dialysis or a transplant. In fibrosis, your kidney tissue doesn't heal as it should, and excess collagen builds up as scar tissue. When scar tissue builds up, your kidneys can't work properly. Damage can be very gradual; in fact, symptoms may not occur until kidney function is less than one-tenth of normal. Both high blood pressure and high salt intakes have been shown to cause renal fibrosis.[19, 20] Twenty-six million Americans have chronic kidney disease (CKD)—defined as some type of kidney problem—and millions of others, including people with hypertension, are at risk of developing CKD.[21]

When the kidneys fail, waste products and excess fluid build up in your body, and you may require dialysis or a kidney transplant. More than 525,000 Americans had end-stage renal disease (ESRD) in 2007. ESRD is complete (or almost complete) kidney failure. People at this stage need either dialysis or a transplant. It's estimated that almost one-quarter of these cases of ESRD were a result of high blood pressure.[22]

Stroke

STROKE IS THE THIRD LEADING CAUSE of death in America and is one of the leading causes of disability.[23] What causes a stroke? Just like everything else in your body, your brain is fed by blood through arteries. And just as high blood pressure can damage the arteries of your heart, it can damage the arteries leading to your brain. If the arteries to your brain are only partially blocked, you can experience a transient ischemic attack—kind of like a ministroke. It's a brief, temporary disruption of blood to your brain caused by a blood clot or

A Salt Emergency

Usually, the effects of high blood pressure cause gradual damage over time. But in some cases, blood pressure can rise so quickly that it becomes an emergency. Symptoms of a high blood pressure emergency include headache, seizure, chest pain, shortness of breath, or edema (fluid buildup in your tissues). This can happen because blood pressure isn't adequately controlled, and it can lead to severe health issues, including:

- **Heart attack**
- **Stroke**
- **Angina,** or unstable chest pain
- **Acute renal failure,** or sudden loss of kidney function
- **Pulmonary edema,** which is when fluid backs up in the lungs and causes shortness of breath
- **Preeclampsia,** a serious condition in pregnancy that can lead to seizures and may require immediate delivery of the baby
- **Encephalopathy,** which includes problems with the brain such as memory loss and personality changes and can progress to dementia, seizures, and coma
- **Aortic dissection,** which is serious damage to the aorta, the main artery of the heart

atherosclerosis. A *stroke* is a longer disruption of blood flow to your brain. Oxygen and nutrients are stopped from entering your brain, causing brain cells to die.

Excess sodium leads to high blood pressure, which can cause a stroke by weakening the blood vessels of the brain.[24] A study commissioned by the World Health Organization showed that increased blood pressure was found to be the largest contributor to stroke, accounting for 62 percent of strokes.[25] People with normal blood pressure (less than 120/80 mmHg) have about half the lifetime risk of stroke compared to people with high blood pressure.[26] Again, just a small reduction in salt intake—as little as 5 grams fewer per day—can lead to a 23 percent lower rate of strokes.[27]

Dementia

HIGH BLOOD PRESSURE caused by consuming too much salt can also affect your thinking.[28] *Dementia,* a loss of brain function that affects memory, thinking, language, judgment, and behavior, can be caused by the narrowing or blockage of the brain's blood vessels, and 14 percent of all people age 71 and over suffer from this disorder.[29] There is evidence that hypertension raises the risk of dementia. In the Women's Health Initiative Memory Study, which took MRI brain scans of 1,400 women over age 65, those with high blood pressure had more abnormal brain lesions 8 years later.[30] Other studies have shown that people with high blood pressure are up to 600 percent more likely to develop vascular, or stroke-related, dementia.[31]

Thus, reducing salt intake and lowering blood pressure can reduce your risk of developing dementia. Researchers have shown that treating hypertension can reduce dementia resulting from Alzheimer's disease by half.[32] Maybe your forgetfulness isn't because you're getting older. It could be caused by how much salt you eat!

Diabetes

D IABETES IS A CHRONIC CONDITION that's marked by high levels of sugar in the blood. It affects more than 20 million Americans, and 40 million more people have prediabetes, which means they have higher than normal levels of blood sugar and a higher chance of developing diabetes. Diabetes can be caused by too little insulin, a resistance of the body's cells to insulin, or both. Insulin, a hormone produced by the pancreas, moves sugar from the blood into the body's cells. Type 1 diabetes is usually diagnosed in childhood and occurs when the body produces little or no insulin. The cause of type 1 diabetes is unknown, but it's most likely genetic in nature.

Type 2 diabetes is more common than type 1 and occurs because the pancreas cannot produce enough insulin to control blood sugar levels or because the body has stopped responding to insulin. In fact, 90 percent of people with type 2 diabetes have a decreased ability to respond to the effects of insulin, and studies indicate that a high-salt diet may be a factor promoting insulin resistance.[33] Unlike type 1 diabetes, type 2 is caused by controllable risk factors, including obesity, lack of exercise, and diet.

Diabetes already puts a person at higher risk for hypertension and heart disease, and a high salt intake will only make these risks greater. People with diabetes have lower blood pressure goals than people without diabetes (130/80 mmHg versus 140/90 mmHg). Controlling blood pressure in people with diabetes is particularly critical because hypertension is an important risk factor for the development and worsening of many complications of diabetes, including diabetic eye disease and kidney disease. Researchers have also found that a higher salt intake is associated with an increased risk of type 2 diabetes.[34]

As we mentioned in Chapter 1, studies in animals show that a high salt intake increases the insulin levels in blood.[35] Since one cause of diabetes is too little insulin in blood, that might seem like it would be a good thing. But too much insulin is also a problem. When you have more insulin than you need to move sugar from the blood into the body's cells, you store more fat and gain more weight.

Metabolic Syndrome

METABOLIC SYNDROME IS CHARACTERIZED by a constellation of symptoms, including abdominal fat, high blood pressure, and high cholesterol. An estimated 50 million Americans have metabolic syndrome.[36] Together, these symptoms increase the risk for coronary heart disease, stroke, and type 2 diabetes. People with metabolic syndrome may benefit more than others from a low-sodium diet to reduce blood pressure. In one study, reducing salt intake decreased the blood pressure by 9/1 mmHg more, on average, of those with metabolic syndrome than the subjects without metabolic syndrome.[37]

Cancer

CANCER IS THE UNCONTROLLED GROWTH of abnormal cells in the body. It can occur almost everywhere throughout the body, including the brain, bone, skin, and internal organs. Overall, more than 11 million Americans have some form of cancer.[38] Although researchers don't yet know exactly how this happens, salted foods may increase cancer risk. High salt intake has been associated with deaths from stomach cancer in some studies. Bacteria called *Helicobacter pylori* can cause stomach cancer, and scientists think that foods high in salt may irritate the stomach lining, which could then make an *H. pylori* infection more likely to occur.[39] In a study of almost 80,000 Japanese subjects, salted foods were linked to a 15 percent increase in total cancers.[40]

Osteoporosis

MORE THAN 44 MILLION AMERICANS have *osteoporosis,* or low bone mass.[41] High-salt diets have been shown to increase calcium loss. When your bones lose calcium, they become weak. Over time, this leads to osteoporosis. Researchers have found that, on average, for every 2,300 milligrams of sodium you ingest, you excrete about 20 to 60 more milligrams of calcium.[42] Researchers think that your body then leeches calcium from your bones to replace the calcium lost and to keep your blood calcium levels stable. A 2-year study conducted in postmenopausal women showed that the amount of loss in hip bone density of patients was related to the amount of sodium subjects ate.[43]

Sleep Apnea

SLEEP APNEA, OR BLOCKED BREATHING when you sleep, occurs more often in people with high blood pressure. It's estimated that approximately 2 percent of American women and 4 percent of American men suffer from sleep apnea. Not only does it cause disrupted sleep, sleep apnea can cause cardiovascular disease from the drops in blood oxygen levels. After many of these low blood oxygen events, sudden death may occur from a heart attack. People with sleep apnea may have two to three times the risk of having high blood pressure than people without sleep apnea. New research also shows that hypertension may actually trigger sleep apnea. It's a vicious cycle—sleep apnea may cause sleep deprivation, which can independently increase blood pressure.

Erectile Dysfunction

LOOD VESSELS BRING BLOOD to your brain, legs, arms, lungs, as well as your sexual organs. Narrowing of these blood vessels caused by sodium-induced high blood pressure can cause erectile dysfunction in men. The likelihood of erectile dysfunction increases with age; studies have found a prevalence of almost 40 percent in 40-year-old men and almost 70 percent in 70-year-old men.[44] Researchers have found that among men with high blood pressure, almost 70 percent are likely to have some form of erectile dysfunction. Another reason to avoid developing hypertension: Erectile dysfunction is a common side effect of medications used to treat high blood pressure.

How the Salt Solution Can Help

OW YOU KNOW THE DANGEROUS EFFECTS of a high-salt diet and how important it is to reduce your sodium intake. Of course, your sodium intake isn't the only factor that can increase your risk of developing high blood pressure, heart disease, diabetes, stroke, or any of the other serious health conditions we've discussed in this chapter.

Let's review some of the other major risk factors for these diseases. You're off the hook on the first set of risk factors—you can't control these.

Age: Your risk of high blood pressure, heart disease, stroke, and diabetes increases as you age. Through early middle age, men are more likely than women to have hypertension. Women are more likely to develop high blood pressure, heart disease, stroke, and diabetes after menopause.

Race: High blood pressure is more common in blacks and often develops earlier than it does in whites. Stroke, heart attacks, and other serious complications are also more common in blacks.

Genetics: Blame your relatives, but unfortunately, high blood pressure and heart disease tend to run in families.

The following risk factors, however, you can control, and the Salt Solution helps you do so.

Being overweight or obese: When you weigh more, you need more blood to circulate throughout your body. As the volume of blood in your body increases, so does blood pressure. Being overweight or obese is also an independent risk factor for heart disease and type 2 diabetes. As we've seen, the Salt Solution can help you lose weight by reducing your cravings for high-fat salty foods and high-calorie sugary drinks.

Being inactive: Being inactive results in higher heart rates, which means your heart has to work harder to pump blood through your body. Hence, you're at higher risk for high blood pressure, heart disease, and diabetes. Inactive people are also more likely to be overweight. Fortunately, the Salt Solution offers an easy exercise program to get you moving.

Smoking: Using tobacco immediately raises blood pressure, but it also causes longer-term effects. Chemicals in tobacco can damage the lining of your artery walls, causing them to narrow. Narrower arteries mean increased risk of high blood pressure, heart disease, and stroke.

Too much alcohol: Drinking too much can damage your heart over time. When you drink more than two or three drinks in a sitting, your blood pressure temporarily increases. Since alcohol is high in calories and lowers your self-control over what you eat, restricting alcohol, as we ask you to do on the Salt Solution, can also help you lose weight.

Not enough potassium in your diet: Potassium balances sodium in your body's cells. Without enough potassium, sodium will escape into your bloodstream, increasing your blood volume, your blood pressure, and your risk of heart disease, diabetes, and stroke. In addition to lowering sodium, the Salt Solution boosts the amount of potassium you eat.

Stress: When you're under stress, your blood pressure can temporarily increase. Common stress relievers such as food, alcohol, and tobacco can also increase your blood pressure, both short- and long-term. Instead, the Salt Solution offers healthy stress-relieving activities like exercise and mindfulness.

Certain chronic conditions: If you have high cholesterol, diabetes, kidney disease, or sleep apnea, your risk of hypertension increases. In a vicious cycle, hypertension in turn increases your risk of developing diabetes, kidney disease, and sleep apnea. The Salt Solution helps break that cycle by lowering sodium intake.

The good news is you can help prevent the damage caused by too much sodium, reduce your risk factors for disease, and drop pounds by making some simple diet changes! Our testers improved many aspects of their health. Most had a significant increase in energy and decrease in blood pressure. Many reported sleeping better and improved moods and self-esteem. One completely rid herself of her bothersome pressure headaches, and another dramatically improved her blood sugar numbers. Cholesterol and triglyceride numbers also improved for some, and one panelist felt so good after the Salt Solution, she finally had the motivation to stop smoking! A strong body of research supports living the Salt Solution way, and in Chapter 3 we'll show you just how easy it is to slash the salt, improve your health, and slim down—forever.

Salt Solution Success Story

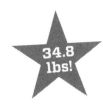

34.8 lbs!

Mark Fatzinger

Age: 39

Pounds Lost: 34.8

Inches Lost: 8³/₄ overall

AS A BUSY MIDDLE SCHOOL GERMAN TEACHER, Mark Fatzinger used to eat on the run, grabbing whatever high-salt, unhealthy foods he could find. His diet relied on vending machine snacks, fast-food value meals, and movie theater popcorn and nachos. As you might expect, he was unhappy with his weight and felt tired all the time.

Mark had tried other diets in the past, but nothing worked for him the way the Salt Solution did. And work it did—in 6 weeks, Mark lost a whopping 35 pounds! What surprised Mark most about the Salt Solution was how much he started wanting to make healthier food choices. "I'm so surprised how much my body lets me know if I make a bad choice now. I enjoy my food more and eat less."

Mark admits, "The Cleanse was painful. Those first 2 weeks were tough. But the plus side was the significant weight loss I saw and how much better I felt." And he says that since the Cleanse recipes were so simple and quick to prepare, it was easy for him to get into the habit of cooking his own meals. Now, he's in the pattern of shopping for fresh healthy food and has gained confidence in the kitchen.

After 6 weeks, Mark sees tons of other benefits besides weight loss from following the Salt Solution. He finds that he's spending a lot less money on food because he is cooking at home rather than going out to eat, and his energy has gone through the roof. "Now I can give my students in my seventh class of the day the same level of enthusiasm I give the students in my first class of the day. And instead of going right home after work, I have the energy to hit the gym a few times a week." Mark says his blood sugar levels are the best they've been in years. In fact, he no longer needs insulin!

SALT SOLUTION MAKEOVER

Mark's "**Before**" Diet

- **BREAKFAST:** 2 doughnuts
- **LUNCH:** Deli Italian sandwich, chicken noodle soup, potato chips, and diet soda
- **DINNER:** Fast-food value meal (cheeseburger, fries, diet soda) and chicken nuggets
- **SNACK:** Diet soda, buttered popcorn

Mark's "**After**" Diet

- **BREAKFAST:** Cranberries-on-a-Banana
- **SNACK:** Banana-Spinach Smoothie
- **LUNCH:** Mini eggplant pizza and spinach salad
- **DINNER:** Indian-Style Chicken
- **SNACK:** Orange-Yogurt Pop and almonds

"**Before**" Nutrition

- **Calories:** 3,058
- **Sodium:** 7,218 mg
- **Saturated Fat:** 49 g
- **Fiber:** 22 g

"**After**" Nutrition

- **Calories:** 1,471
- **Sodium:** 919 mg
- **Saturated Fat:** 8 g
- **Fiber:** 27 g

Salt Solution Improvements: With the Salt Solution, Mark is now eating about eight times less salt (7,218 mg versus 919 mg). He also has drastically reduced his caloric intake (3,058 to 1,471 calories). Before the Salt Solution, the only fresh vegetables Mark ate were the lettuce and tomato on a fast-food cheeseburger. Now he buys fresh fruits and vegetables, whole grains, and lean proteins, and he enjoys cooking for himself. You can see the difference in Mark's weight and the inches he's lost, but there are hidden improvements—after 6 weeks of the Salt Solution, Mark's blood pressure dropped from 130/90 mmHg to 120/80 mmHg, now within the healthy range.

SODIUM, THE SILENT KILLER

The Salt

SOLUTION

LOWDOWN

Shake the salt and you'll lose weight and feel better. It's just that simple. Study after study (after study after study!) has shown that lowering salt intake reduces the risk of chronic disease, prevents death, and improves health. In fact, researchers recently calculated that 8.5 million deaths could be prevented over a 10-year period with only a 15 percent decrease in salt intake.[1] For the average American, that's just slightly more than 500 milligrams of sodium (about ¼ teaspoon of table salt), less than the amount you'd find in a few slices of deli ham. Researchers at the University of California, San Francisco, Stanford University, and Columbia University calculated that if Americans reduced their sodium intake by 1,200 milligrams per day, or about ½ teaspoon of table salt—described by researchers as "hardly detectable" in terms of the taste of food—it would reduce the annual number of new cases of coronary heart disease by 60,000, stroke by 32,000, heart attack by 54,000, and the annual number of deaths by 44,000. In addition to this massive benefit in the health of Americans, a small salt intake reduction like this would result in $24 billion worth of savings in health care costs.[2]

Reducing salt may be more important to your health than other dietary changes! By making a few easy changes and by getting back to eating real foods with real flavors, you'll improve your health, drop pounds, and enjoy eating more than ever. We'll show you just how simple it is to clean out your diet and slash the salt.

How to Go Low Salt

THE SOLUTION IS the Salt Solution! The Salt Solution Diet isn't about deprivation. It's about what you can eat as opposed to what you should not eat. The Salt Solution contains just the right mix of vitamins, minerals, protein, fiber—and flavor, so you'll lose salt but not taste. With the Salt Solution, you'll reduce your sodium to no more than 1,500 milligrams per day, but it's not only reducing sodium that's important. Increasing the amount of potassium, calcium, and magnesium is also critical.[3, 4] While our current sodium intake far exceeds recommended levels, by contrast, our intake of these important minerals is remarkably low.

Miracle Minerals

Researchers have found that increasing your intake of potassium, calcium, and magnesium helps to counteract the negative effects of sodium and balance your mineral levels.[5] Here's the lowdown on these Miracle Minerals.

Potassium: This mineral is involved in nerve function, muscle control, and blood pressure. Potassium is essential in the transport of neural impulses and the movement of muscles. When you pull your hand away from a hot stove, potassium helps tell your brain that you're getting burned. And just as sodium can increase blood pressure, potassium can lower it. Potassium and sodium work together to regulate the body's water balance. Potassium increases the amount of sodium excreted from the body, and, as you know, the less sodium, the better. Potassium may also protect against stroke and other cardiovascular disease, including the development of atherosclerosis, or plaque, in your arteries. Adults should eat 4,700 milligrams of potassium per day, but most Americans eat less than half the recommended amount. Can you just take a pill? Nope. It's much better to get potassium from foods you eat (see "Should I supplement?"). It's found at high levels in many fruits, vegetables, and beans—healthy foods

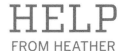
FROM HEATHER

Should I supplement?

The best way to get what your body needs is in food, not pills. In fact, scientists have discovered it is impossible to reproduce the beneficial interactions that occur between nutrients and foods by just taking a pill. The Salt Solution provides you with all the necessary nutrients from the best possible source: food. However, since eating an optimum diet every day is not always possible, it's a good idea to take a daily multivitamin/mineral pill. But remember, more is not always better, and taking megadoses of any vitamin or mineral (even the Miracle Minerals) is not only a waste of money but also a source of potential harm. Look for multis with no more than 100 percent of the Daily Value of each vitamin and mineral it contains. Taking this amount in a daily won't put you at risk for overdoing it on the Salt Solution. Dietary supplements are not required to undergo the same testing as medicines, so choose well-known mainstream brands and buy from large, trusted retailers.

you should be eating more of. The Salt Solution program contains many foods that are rich in potassium and low in sodium.

Calcium: This mineral also increases sodium excretion. It is found in dairy products and some vegetables. Studies have shown that supplementation with calcium lowers blood pressure. Adults need between 1,000 and 1,300 milligrams of calcium per day, depending on their age, but most Americans get only about 35 to 40 percent of this recommendation. You'll be getting your calcium in the Salt Solution program from low-fat and fat-free dairy items. Besides being lower in calories, low-fat and fat-free dairy products actually have more calcium than their high-fat relatives! Because calcium in dairy products is not contained in the fat portion of these products, removing fat increases the amount of calcium that's in a given volume of the dairy product. In order to get all the benefits of calcium, you need to have plenty of vitamin D, and most dairy products are fortified with it. There's an added bonus in all the calcium you'll get in the Salt Solution program: Increased calcium intake can also improve bone health and prevent osteoporosis, and can also help speed weight loss and prevent weight gain. As with potassium, although you can supplement your calcium intake with vitamins, it's best to focus on whole food sources of calcium as your first line of defense.

Magnesium: This is the most abundant mineral in the human body. In fact, more than 300 biochemical processes in your body depend on magnesium. It's necessary for muscle and nerve function and for blood sugar regulation, as magnesium may increase the excretion of insulin, which regulates the body's blood sugar. Some studies have shown that lower magnesium intake is linked to higher risk of developing diabetes.[6] We know that increased magnesium intake increases sodium excretion. Some researchers think it plays a role in relaxing blood vessels, which can lower blood pressure. Chances are, if you're like most Americans, you're getting about half as much magnesium as you should. The recommended dietary allowance for magnesium is 310 to 420 milligrams per day, depending on age and sex. If you eat a wide variety of beans, nuts, whole grains, and vegetables—which you'll be doing when you follow the Salt Solution program—you'll be getting plenty of this valuable mineral.

Although there are lots of other minerals that are important to your health (and the Salt Solution provides you with all the nutrients you need for optimum health), we're focusing on potassium, calcium, and magnesium because these Miracle Minerals can help counter the negative effects of sodium—high blood pressure, heart attack, stroke, kidney disease, dementia, diabetes, metabolic syndrome, osteoporosis, cancer, and, of course, weight gain. As with any minerals, it's important to keep them in balance. There are side effects to getting too much of the Miracle Minerals, but if you're a healthy adult, you can't get too much potassium, calcium, or magnesium from eating foods and/or a regular multivitamin. If you are taking extra supplements of these minerals, consult your doctor (see "Should I supplement?" on page 43).

THE SALT SOLUTION STARS

So how can you be sure to get enough of these Miracle Minerals? Not to worry. The Salt Solution eating plan features the mineral-loaded Salt Solution Stars. They're all excellent sources of either calcium, potassium, or magnesium, and many are great sources of all three!

★ **BANANAS:** Packed with potassium, bananas are Salt Solution staples. More good banana news: They're also chockful of vitamin B$_6$, filling fiber, and vitamin C.

★ **BEET GREENS:** These root vegetable greens are full of potassium, magnesium, and calcium! A true Salt Solution superfood, beet greens are also loaded with vitamin K and beta-carotene.

★ **HALIBUT:** This high-quality protein source is brimming with magnesium and potassium. It's also low in heart-harming saturated fats and high in heart-healthy omega-3 fatty acids, making this fish a Salt Solution win-win.

★ **KALE:** Full of not only calcium and potassium, but also iron and vitamins A and C, including this nutrient-dense leafy green in your diet is a surefire way to boost your health.

★ **MILK:** Milk really does do a body good! It's a convenient source of calcium, and it's loaded with protein and fortified with vitamins D and A. Just be sure to choose low-fat or fat-free milk to reduce the bad-for-you fat found in whole milk.

★ **SARDINES:** These tiny fish pack a powerful potassium and calcium punch and are loaded with omega-3 fatty acids and protein. Canned low-sodium sardines are an affordable and tasty Salt Solution pantry staple.

★ **SOYBEANS:** Rich in calcium, potassium, and magnesium, soybeans are nutritional powerhouses. Whether fresh, roasted, or dried, this wonder veggie is also rich in iron, zinc, and lots of B vitamins. (Young soybeans are also known as edamame.)

★ **SOYMILK:** Soymilk is rich in potassium and magnesium, and if you pick up a calcium-fortified brand like Silk, you'll be getting as much of this important mineral as you'd find in cow's milk.

★ **SPINACH:** Popeye was no fool. Crammed with potassium, magnesium, and calcium as well as vitamins A and C and folate, spinach is a nutrient-packed Salt Solution superfood.

★ **SWEET POTATOES:** Like the banana, these root veggies are an excellent source of potassium. They're also a rich source of antioxidants, including vitamin C and beta-carotene. Eat the skin and you'll also get a hefty dose of fill-you-up fiber.

★ **WHITE BEANS:** These legumes are packed not only with protein, fiber, and iron, but also potassium, magnesium, and calcium. They're a 3-in-1 Salt Solution must-have.

★ **YOGURT:** Most of us know this dairy snack is loaded with calcium, but did you know it's also a good source of potassium and magnesium? Yup, it's true. Just be sure to stick with low-fat or fat-free varieties to limit bad-for-your-heart saturated fat.

If some of these foods are unfamiliar to you, don't worry. We'll give you plenty of ideas for how to prepare them in the recipes in Chapter 6. Also, we've identified these Salt Solution Stars as some of the best sources of our Miracle Minerals, but they are by no means the only sources. See the Appendix: Where to Find the Miracle Minerals on page 284 for a complete list of foods high in calcium, potassium, and magnesium.

Beyond the Miracle Minerals

WHAT ELSE WILL YOU BE EATING on the Salt Solution diet? Whole, unprocessed foods, including whole grains, lots of fresh fruits and vegetables, low-fat or fat-free dairy, healthy fats, lean meats, poultry, and fish. You'll find that after you start eating clean, whole foods, you'll most likely lose your taste for processed foods chockful of preservatives and additives. Not to worry, though, you won't have to eat an expensive and restrictive organic-only diet. On the other hand, we have nothing against eating organic. It is better for the environment and reduces your exposure to potentially dangerous chemicals. But certain organic foods have more impact than others. To get the most organic (and Salt Solution) bang for your buck, check out "Understanding Organic" on page 198.

You'll never feel deprived on the Salt Solution. You'll be enjoying the delicious food so much you'll never miss the salt! This will make sticking with the Salt Solution plan something you'll want to do, not something you're forced to do.

The Salt Solution meals are structured around five major components: protein, dairy, produce, grains, and fat. In addition to the general guidelines we give here about finding low-sodium foods in each of these categories, Chapter 7 gives lists of specific low-sodium brands to look for.

Protein Power

Proteins are made of chains of molecules called *amino acids,* which are essential for building and repairing muscle. What makes protein so great? It takes your body longer to digest protein than to digest simple carbohydrates, so protein helps keep you feeling full for longer. Eating protein can even help boost your metabolism, because it takes our bodies three times more energy to digest protein than to digest carbs or fat. More energy expended by your body equals more calories burned.

Adults need a minimum of 0.8 gram of protein for every kilogram of body weight daily, or just about 8 grams of protein for every 20 pounds of body weight.[7] You'll want to make sure that you're getting enough protein, but like anything you eat, too much is not a good thing. Just like too many carbohydrates or too much fat, if you eat too much protein, it will be stored as fat. Another thing to remember is that you want to focus on lean meats to meet your protein needs rather than on fatty red meats. Lean proteins like fish, chicken breast, pork tenderloin, turkey, or seafood are lower in saturated fat and are featured in the Salt Solution. Eating too much red meat has been associated with health risks such as increased cholesterol, heart attack, stroke, and certain cancers.[8] Don't eat meat at all? No problem. Just choose smart Salt Solution veggie options like tofu and other soy products as well as beans, nuts, eggs, and nut butters and you'll get all the protein you need.

Natural, minimally processed meats like chicken breast or pork tenderloin are naturally low in sodium. Problems start when you head to the deli counter or prepared meats section, where you'll find both meats and protein products that have been pumped with sodium. You'll see how important it is to read labels. Products that look the same can actually have widely different sodium contents.

Why do some items vary so much? Many producers sell "enhanced" meat that has been injected with or soaked in a salt solution broth to keep it moist and improve its flavor. Most enhanced chickens have two to three times higher sodium levels than nonenhanced cluckers, and enhanced pork can have up to five times higher levels. Check the ingredient list for sodium or salt and check the product label for words like "self-basting" or "percent solution" or "broth," all terms that indicate that salt may have been added. Keep in mind that raw meat contains some naturally occurring sodium. For example, an ounce of chicken contains about 20 milligrams of naturally occurring sodium, so a 4-ounce breast starts out with 80 milligrams of sodium before it's injected. (See page 198 for more on buying meat and eggs directly from local ranchers through community sustainable agriculture, or CSA, groups.)

Dairy Delivers

Dairy products are essential for bone health, blood pressure control, and weight loss. We know that calcium keeps bones healthy and lowers blood pressure and that dairy products are great sources of calcium. As we mentioned earlier in the chapter, calcium increases sodium excretion. But how does it help you lose weight? One study found that people who followed a diet that included

800 milligrams of calcium supplements lost significantly more weight than those who had only about half that amount of calcium in their diets; those who had gotten their calcium through dairy products (3 servings a day, or about 1,200 to 1,300 milligrams of calcium) lost even more weight.[9] Some studies have found that adults who eat a high-dairy diet have lost significantly more weight and fat than those who consume a low-dairy diet containing the same number of calories.[10] Researchers aren't sure exactly why, but they think that dietary calcium may increase fat burning and decrease fat storage. Pass the yogurt!

In order for calcium to have the best effects, it should be combined with vitamin D. Your body needs an adequate amount of vitamin D to absorb calcium. This is why milk and other dairy products are fortified with vitamin D and why calcium supplements have vitamin D added. (If your supplement doesn't, choose a different one.)

To get the best benefits from dairy, the Salt Solution sticks to low-fat and fat-free choices, like fat-free milk, yogurt, cottage and ricotta cheese, and other types of reduced-fat cheeses. Full-fat milk and cheeses do have the benefits of calcium, but they also come with tons of fat and calories. As mentioned earlier, low-fat and fat-free dairy products usually have more calcium than their high-fat relatives! And, of course, we steer you away from higher-sodium dairy choices like most processed cheeses and buttermilk.

How do you pick the best dairy products? Read the labels, and look for the sodium. There are low-salt options for most of your favorite dairy items.

Pump Up the Produce

Fruits and veggies are Salt Solution superfoods. Although some fruits and vegetables contain sodium naturally (and that's okay!), the overall amount of sodium in fresh produce is low, and they are packed with essential vitamins, minerals, and fiber, are low in saturated fats, and they taste delicious. Fruits and vegetables are full of compounds called phytochemicals and antioxidants, which may help slow down the aging process and reduce the risk of many diseases, such as cancer, heart disease, stroke, high blood pressure, osteoporosis, urinary tract infections, and cataracts.[11]

How do you know which fruits and veggies are best? Look for the Salt Solution Stars (see page 45), of course, as they're loaded with minerals that help counteract the negative effects of sodium, and aim for color. Phytochemicals are usually related to plant pigments, so bright-colored fruits and veggies—like yellow, orange, red, green, blue, and purple—are nutrient packed. Try to choose the freshest produce available. To follow the Salt Solution plan, you'll want to steer clear of canned fruits and vegetables, which are generally very high in salt. Eat foods in season, check out your local farmers' markets, and ask employees at your local grocery store. Can't get to the farm stand for fresh produce? Frozen fruits and vegetables are generally low in sodium and a good backup plan. Just make sure to check the labels before you buy. Pick products with no added sodium, and stay away from veggies that are frozen with a flavored sauce. (See page 198 for more on buying produce directly from local farms through CSA groups.)

Get Your Grains

Yes, grains are carbohydrates, but regardless of the myth that carbs make you fat, not all carbohydrates are bad. In fact, carbohydrates are absolutely essential for energy. What's the difference between good and bad carbs? In general, the longer a carbohydrate takes to break down in the body, the better it is. These carbs keep you feeling full longer and generally contain more vitamins, minerals, and fiber. Simple carbs, like white bread and rice, are digested very quickly. Complex carbohydrates, found in whole grains like processed whole wheat bread, oatmeal, and brown rice, take longer for the body to break down and digest.

In addition to keeping you feeling fuller longer, whole grains are also healthier. They're a better source of fiber and the good-for-your-health minerals potassium and magnesium.[12] A diet high in whole grains like the Salt Solution has been linked with a lower risk of cardiovascular disease as well as type 2 diabetes and cancer.[13] Eating whole grains may also be related to weight loss. One 12-year study found that women who consistently consumed more whole grains weighed less than women who consumed fewer whole grains; those who ate the most fiber had a lower risk of major weight gain.[14] Another study, this one in men, showed that eating whole grains and bran were independently related to less weight gain.[15]

Stick with plain, unflavored grains to stay low in salt, and make sure to check the sodium content before you buy. (Plain doesn't mean boring. Add fresh herbs or your favorite salt-free dried seasonings to spice up your grains!)

Fill Up with Fats

Fats do not necessarily make you fat. You need to eat some fat to absorb certain vitamins, and fats are essential for energy. The problem begins when we eat too much fat and it's stored in our bodies. As we mentioned earlier, scientists have discovered that some combos of fatty and salty foods, like salted and buttered popcorn, for example, have a high capacity to intensify appetite. Brain scans show that these types of foods cause the brain to release *dopamine,* the neurotransmitter associated with the pleasure center, making them addictive and hard to resist. So although you need to include fat in your diet, just like with protein and carbohydrates, the type of fat and foods you eat matters.

In general, plant-based fats are healthier than meat-based fats. Plant-based fats—like those found in avocados, nuts, seeds, and olive oil—are recommended on the Salt Solution as they are lower in saturated fat (the "bad" fat) than meat-based fats like those found in beef, bacon, and butter.

Even worse than saturated fats are trans fats, which have been shown to increase heart disease risk. Trans fats are found in partially hydrogenated oils, stable oils that help keep foods fresh longer. Where will you see these? In fried items and packaged foods like cookies and crackers, which also happen to have the addictive qualities you want to avoid. Check the labels, and avoid anything with trans fats in the Nutrition Facts panel or partially hydrogenated oils or shortening in the ingredients list. Avoid other fat-and-salt-packed items that run the risk of being dangerously addictive—foods like salted nuts, chips, cheese puffs, snack cakes, pies, and pastries.

Want to get the most flavorful low-salt fats for your calorie buck? Stick with unsalted, natural items—unsalted butter, peanut butter and other nut butters, unsalted nuts, and pure olive and vegetable oils.

Real Life; Real Results

When we created the Salt Solution program, we knew it was a winning combo that would help people improve their health and lose weight because it's a nonfad approach based on the latest scientific research. But we were eager to put it into action and see real results with real people just like you. So we recruited a test panel of 16 men and women who were ready to break their salt habit and make some healthy lifestyle changes.

Some were very aware of their addiction to salt and ready to make a change. They admitted to salting without tasting, upping the sodium in their everyday recipes, and eating an abundance of overly salted processed and fast foods. One even carried a mini saltshaker in her purse "just in case." Others were less concerned with sodium and more worried about the extra pounds they had been carrying around for a few years and, for some, a few decades. They were giving the Salt Solution a whirl in hopes that a reduction in salt would also mean a reduction in weight. Some had never lost the baby weight, while others had gained the weight due to a stressful job or a family crisis. Some had been accumulating the pounds slowly one year (and one pound) at a time, and still others were just having a hard time balancing the

demands of family, work, and their own health needs. One had recently lost a lot of weight but hoped the Salt Solution would help her improve her overall health and increase her energy levels.

BREAKING THE SALT ADDICTION
While their motivations and situations were different, their Salt Solution experiences were similar—and inspiring! They all broke their dependence on salt and dropped pounds and inches—Mark Fatzinger, a 39-year-old middle school teacher, lost an astonishing 34.8 pounds and $8^3/_4$ inches in just 6 weeks of the Salt Solution! "I'm more aware of how food impacts how I feel. Now, when I could have made a better food choice, I feel it. And I much prefer feeling good."

Robin Scholtz, 45, who lost a total of 14.8 pounds and $12^1/_4$ inches, says, "I feel better and look better than I have in years." A store manager who has had trouble with her weight since childhood, she explained, "I have struggled with my weight all my life! I was a chubby kid and it only got worse after I got pregnant with my daughter. Now, with help from the Salt Solution, my self-esteem is up. Although the first 2 weeks of the plan were a challenge, it was well worth it! I feel like a new person, and I don't even miss the salt! The Cleanse totally changed my taste for food."

Like Robin, other participants found that their taste buds were transformed by the 2-Week Cleanse. "After about 5 days, my salt cravings ended, and my sugar cravings and compulsive eating stopped, too," says Laura Gutierrez, a 47-year-old manager. Shannon Ferry, a 35-year-old teacher, explains, "I have not added salt to my food since I began this plan. My husband and I both would always have the saltshaker within reach during our meals, even though I would add salt during the cooking process. Since I started this plan, my salt cravings became nonexistent, and if I tasted something that did have salt, it always tasted way too salty."

DISCOVERING NEW FLAVORS

Many panelists reported that their "palate expanded" and that they could "actually taste again." Some found unsalted foods more gratifying. "I discovered that certain foods like nuts, when eaten without salt, are not as addictive and seem more satisfying," says Gloria Greech, a 57-year-old legal secretary.

Test panelists unanimously enjoyed the foods on the Salt Solution program. "I loved that the plan was all real food! Our refrigerator and pantry is filled with fruits, veggies, nuts, and other fresh things," says Laura. "Because I actually liked the recipes and felt full after eating them, it didn't seem like I was 'dieting.' It was the perfect amount," explains Shannon. "I've discovered a lot of new spices and flavors and that, when I use these, I don't even miss the salt," says Gretchen Tonno, a 49-year-old marketing manager.

Other panelists found that they loved cooking their own food. "I was afraid of cooking," says Mark. "The plan helped to establish patterns of shopping for fresh healthy food, using it and not letting it spoil, and generally taking care of myself. I enjoy cooking for myself now, and I'm spending a lot less money on food."

SLEUTHING OUT SODIUM

Most panelists had no idea how much sodium they were consuming before beginning the Salt Solution. Says Diane Anderson, a 58-year-old physical therapist, "I was continually amazed by how much sodium is in food. Food items that I never suspected had salt in them were loaded with sodium!" Michael Tonno shares Diane's sentiments. "Since I never added salt to my food, I never paid attention to the salt content. But now I realize just how much salt I was eating every day."

Melanie Cardell, 37, a sports medicine trainer, had tried lots of diets in the past, but with the Salt Solution, she finally found the missing diet link. "The more I found out and read about the nutritional information of fast food and packaged food, it made me not want to eat it," explains Melanie. "Not just the sodium content is awful, but also the calories and the ingredients. This plan made me way more conscious of the labels and food in general." And the more conscious she became about the foods she ate, the more success she had. "The pounds just dropped off, and the more weight I lost, the more motivated I was to keep losing." Now, 12 pounds lighter, Melanie has started swimming, running, and biking to get into shape. Come 2011, she will participate in her first triathlon.

ENJOYING MORE ENERGY
The panelists collectively reported that their energy levels soared. "I felt light and energetic, and I even slept better," says 68-year-old Denise Battista, a retired schoolteacher.

Alice Mudge, a 60-year-old administrative assistant, used to come home from work and collapse in front of the television, but not anymore. Their increased energy led to an increase in their activity—one started Zumba classes, another doubled the length of her daily dog walks.

Shannon also suffered from a total lack of energy at the end of the workday, which affected her mood. "Since starting the plan, I wake up more refreshed, even though my sleep hours have not changed much. I am more energized throughout the day, and when I come home, I don't need to lie down. I'm also not as cranky as I was before!" Mark also reports feeling better emotionally after participating in the Salt Solution. "I wake up earlier and have more energy throughout the day. This means I'm more patient at work." As a middle school teacher, we know Mark needs lots of patience!

IMPROVING HEALTH
While losing pounds and inches and gaining energy, test panelists also improved their general well-being. As blood pressure numbers dropped, their overall health (and attitudes!)

improved. "I can't wait to jump out of bed and get my day going," explains Dianne Daniels, a 47-year-old administrative assistant. "Before, I used to experience 'blue days' where it was an effort to even get out of bed. Since detoxing from salt using the Salt Solution, I'm much more energetic, I don't find myself falling asleep halfway through the day, and I don't have headaches anymore. I used to see 'floaters' and have flashes of light—symptoms of high blood pressure, which ran in my family. Now my blood pressure is down, and I look and feel fantastic."

Others improved their blood sugar numbers; in fact, Mark's blood sugar is so much better, he no longer has to take insulin! Some participants, like Melanie, significantly improved their cholesterol and triglyceride numbers. One was feeling so wonderful on the Salt Solution plan, she quit smoking!

MAKING THE CHANGES LAST
While the results of the test panel were certainly encouraging, we were even more pleased with the panelists' attitudes toward making these changes stick for life. Shannon notes, "I have learned that food is my fuel, and in order to get myself going, I need to eat good things." She used to feel uncomfortable with her appearance and felt that she wasn't a good role model for her students. Now everything's changed. "I plan to continue following this lifestyle, changing my habits and mind-set about food and eating. I have the knowledge that I need to be healthy!"

Perhaps the best part about the Salt Solution being a lifelong process is that our panelists realized they could share it with their loved ones. "My whole family has been very supportive," explains Beth Vorosmarti, a 47-year-old homemaker and artist. "My kids are eating more fresh fruit than they might have otherwise. We are all reading labels for sodium content. My son was especially surprised about ketchup, which he used to use all the time." Michael and Gretchen Tonno were both panelists and lost a combined 28 pounds and 11 inches after 6 weeks of the Salt Solution! Says Mike, "My wife and I cook and exercise together. It is fun and making us an even stronger couple."

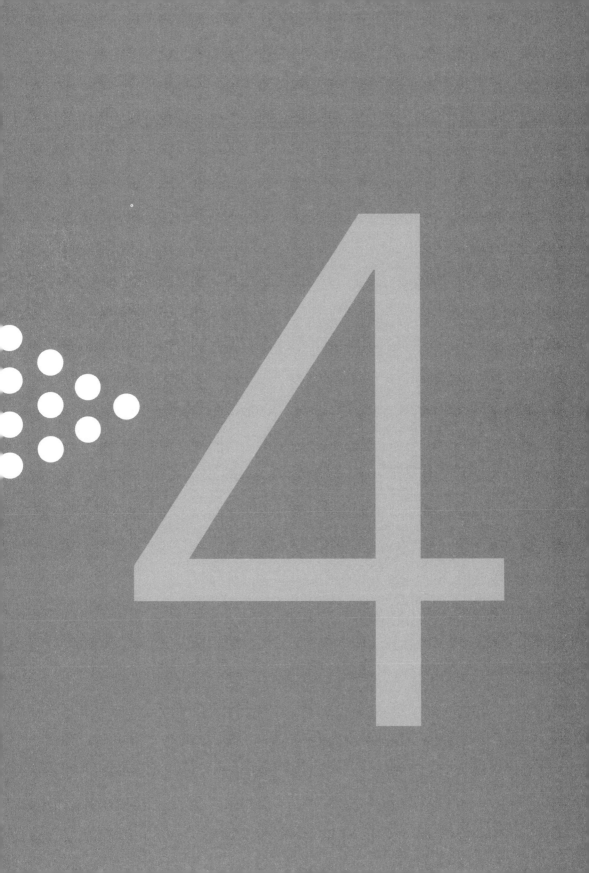

THE 2-WEEK Salt SOLUTION CLEANSE

Okay, everyone, it's time to clean up your diet, drop pounds, and start living the Salt Solution way! The 2-Week Salt Solution Cleanse is designed to boost metabolism, increase energy, and cleanse the system of excess sodium, saturated and trans fat, and unnecessary chemicals and substances such as food dyes, artificial sweeteners, and alcohol. The Cleanse will also jump-start weight loss and eliminate bloating caused by salt. In just 2 weeks, you'll drop pounds and lose inches, which will motivate you and set you up for success on the 4-Week Shake the Salt Meal Plan.

The Goals of the 2-Week Cleanse

T HE 2-WEEK CLEANSE HAS BEEN CREATED for the specific purpose of decreasing salt and eliminating toxins in your diet so you will feel and look your best fast! But not to worry. This is not some crazy—and unhealthy—"detox" diet. No way! You'll be eating fruits, vegetables, whole grains, herbs, chicken, fish, and more—in other words, you'll be eating natural, real food. More good news: The Cleanse will not only rid your system of unwanted chemicals, it will also reset your taste buds. And that's a good thing, since most of our taste buds are completely out of whack.

How did they get this way? Processed foods full of chemicals create tastes that don't exist in nature. Think about sour cream and onion potato chips or cheese-flavored crackers. What about fruit-flavored candy? Foods that are produced to taste like the real thing are aggressively flavored; therefore, they taste a whole lot stronger than the actual food they mimic. In addition, packaged foods, fast foods, and many restaurant foods are swimming in sodium. The amount of sodium in an average chain restaurant meal is truly astounding. We're talking five times the amount of sodium you need in a single day, much less in one meal. When your taste buds adjust to these intense flavors and seasoning, food in its natural form can taste bland in comparison.

Luckily, our taste buds are more adaptable than you may think. Most of us have around 10,000 taste buds, and each one is made up of between 50 and 150 receptor cells. Receptor cells live for only 1 to 2 weeks and then are replaced by new cells. So after eating a clean diet for a week or two, your taste buds will adjust and you will begin to taste the subtle flavors in real foods, the way Mother Nature intended. An apple, a berry, or a piece of pineapple actually tastes incredible, as do bell peppers, nuts, honey, and other fresh foods. Overly salted and processed fare can't hold a candle to the real thing! Clear your diet of sodium-laced processed foods and you won't want to go back. That's a promise.

The 2-Week Cleanse won't be easy. You'll be giving up some favorite foods, cutting out alcohol, and eliminating dining out as much as possible, but it'll be worth it! At the end of the 14 days, you'll be slimmer and healthier, and your salt addiction will be a thing of the past. Some of our test panelists lost more than 10 pounds in these 2 weeks! (Shannon Ferry dropped 10.6 pounds and 5 inches; Robin Scholtz lost 10.4 pounds and 4¾ inches.)

And all of the participants were astonished at how painless it was to break their salt habit. "The 2-Week Cleanse was instrumental in breaking my salt habit," says test panelist Dianne Daniels. "I was so encouraged by the taste of the food that after the first couple of days, I didn't miss the salt at all. I used to salt my food without even tasting it. Now I don't even pick up a saltshaker!"

That's not all. The panelists also reported feeling energized and refreshed, and as the pounds peeled off, their motivation picked up. "I was surprised at how much weight I lost during the Cleanse," explains Melanie Cardell. "I felt great. The more weight I lost, the more energy I had, and the more motivated I became to keep going!"

During the 2-Week Cleanse you will:

Purify Your System: Alcohol and processed foods are restricted, and Cleanse meals are based around clean foods with no artificial ingredients. The diet is not only low in sodium but also in excess fat and sugar as well as free from chemicals and artificial flavoring.

Reset Your Taste Buds: We are hardwired to enjoy the taste of fattening and salty foods. Our brain's pleasure center loves foods that are high in salt, sugar, and fat. By cutting out processed items and eating clean, whole foods, you'll reset your taste buds. Soon you'll find high-sodium foods too salty, and you'll crave the naturally delicious flavors of fruits, vegetables, and whole grains.

Reduce Bloating: You know that sodium loves water. The more sodium in your bloodstream, the more water, which leads to extra water weight and a sluggish feeling. You'll decrease bloating and lose the excess water weight by cutting the sodium.

Balance Minerals: For optimum mineral levels and good health, it's important that you not only decrease sodium but also increase potassium, calcium, and magnesium. The meals and the Mineral Boost Juices featured in the 2-Week Cleanse are packed with the Salt Solution Stars, foods high in these Miracle Minerals (see page 42), and will bring your body back into balance.

Speed Weight Loss: The 2-Week Cleanse helps you lose weight in two ways. First, the extra water weight will melt away as you cut salt. Then the low-calorie (but satisfying!) nutrient-dense meals will give you energy without packing on the pounds.

Train Your Brain: Tracking your intake by writing down not only what you're eating but also why you're eating will keep you from deviating from the plan. In fact, *The Salt Solution Journal* (which you can buy at prevention.com/shop) will be your very own diet sleuth and will help you uncover the unconscious habits that could stand in the way of your success.

The 2-Week Cleanse Basics

DURING THE 1,200-CALORIE-A-DAY 2-WEEK CLEANSE, you will eat three 300-calorie meals per day, each featuring a nutrient-packed Salt Solution Star (see page 45) and each with no more than about 300 milligrams of sodium. You will also have a daily 300-calorie Mineral Boost

Juice. Be sure to have a meal or Mineral Boost Juice approximately every 4 to 5 hours. Your body is like a machine that needs frequent refueling, and going longer between meals almost ensures you will overeat. Eating smaller meals several times a day also gets your body used to a regular meal schedule, which you'll continue to follow on the rest of the Salt Solution plan.

Mix & Match Cleanse Meals: Have Three per Day

You'll find 20 different Cleanse meals to choose from starting on page 70. These tasty meals are packed with the perfect mix of protein, carbs, and fat, so you'll lose weight and burn calories more effectively. As previously mentioned, these meals have been created specifically to provide you with the nutrients you need to cleanse and balance your body. Each meal features one or more of the Salt Solution Stars—foods that provide significant amounts of the key beneficial minerals (potassium, magnesium, and calcium)—and each is loaded with fiber to help you feel full.

Because all of the Cleanse meals provide about 300 calories, you can move them around or swap them out at will. For example, a breakfast meal can be eaten for dinner, a snack can be eaten as breakfast, or a lunch meal as a snack. You may repeat meals that you find most enjoyable if you wish, but variety is strongly encouraged. Dessert and snack meals should be limited to no more than one per day as they don't provide the same balanced nutrition as the other meals. Eat the meals exactly as is except for herbs, spices, and other seasonings that you can add as desired (see the Salt Solution Seasoning Guide on page 204). Just steer clear of sauces or dressings that may contain added oil, sugar, salt, and calories. If you find you are still hungry, you can add any of the foods from the Salt Solution Freebies list (see page 64). These "free" foods are nutrient-dense, low-calorie foods you can use to add bulk to your meals without adding calories.

THE SALT SOLUTION FREEBIES

Add any of these foods to your meals as desired. Because they're very low in calories, it's impossible to eat too much of them. Just be sure not to cook them in a lot of oil or add sauces with added calories and/or salt. Preferred cooking methods are steaming, microwaving, roasting, or boiling.

Artichoke hearts	Cauliflower	Radishes
Asparagus	Celery	*Spinach
*Beet greens	Collard greens	String/green beans
Beets	Cucumbers	Tomatoes
Bell peppers	Eggplant	Water chestnuts
Broccoli	*Kale	Zucchini and
Brussels sprouts	Lettuce	summer squash
Cabbage	Mushrooms	
Carrots	Onions	

*Include this Salt Solution Star as often as possible.

Mineral Boost Juice: Have One per Day

A hallmark of this plan is the daily Mineral Boost Juice, a smoothie pumped with calcium, magnesium, and potassium, the minerals that counteract the negative effects of excess sodium. Drinking a Mineral Boost Juice every day in addition to your three Cleanse meals will not only replenish your body with what it needs but also serve as a reminder that you are working hard to decrease your sodium, increase your nutrients, and improve your life. It will keep you focused on the weight-loss task ahead. There are three versions of the Mineral Boost Juice to choose from (see page 69). Test them out and choose the varieties that taste best to you. You can stick with just one flavor or you can mix them up. The choice is yours.

2-WEEK CLEANSE Q & A'S

Before you get started, here are some questions that were frequently asked by our test panelists. Knowing the answers ahead of time will help you achieve optimal success during your 2-Week Cleanse.

Q. **What if I don't like some of the meals in the meal plan?**

A. During the 2-Week Cleanse, you should stick to the 20 Mix & Match Cleanse Meals and should not swap out ingredients in a meal. These meals are carefully designed to give you balanced nutrition in the optimal amount of 1,200 calories daily. With 20 meals to choose from, there is plenty of variety. You may repeat meals that you find most enjoyable if you wish, but variety is encouraged.

Q. **What if I'm allergic to something on the plan?**

A. During the 2-Week Cleanse, you should stick as closely to the plan as possible. However, if you have an allergy, you can swap a similar ingredient within the same food group—such as tomatoes for red peppers or turkey for chicken.

Q. **Is it important for me to measure my food?**

A. Yes. For accuracy, we request that you measure all your food on this plan. Without measuring, it's very easy to accumulate extra calories. For cup and spoon measurements ($\frac{1}{2}$ cup, 1 tablespoon, etc.), be sure to level the top. It takes only an extra minute to measure food.

Q. **What can I drink during the 2-Week Cleanse?**

A. During the Cleanse, it's best to stick with plain water and unsweetened brewed hot and cold green, red, white, black, or herbal tea, and, of course, one Mineral Boost Juice each day. Alcohol is completely forbidden, and coffee consumption should be limited to no more than 1 cup a day. (Black coffee doesn't add calories, but it can irritate your digestive system; any milk or sugar adds calories.)

Q. **Can I eat out on the 2-Week Cleanse?**

A. For the duration of the 2 weeks, it's best to stick with the Cleanse meals. This will yield not only the best weight-loss results but also ensure that you reduce your sodium intake enough to reset your taste buds. Restaurant meals tend to be loaded with sodium, as well as fat and calories. However, if there are one or two work lunches or other events you absolutely can't avoid during the Cleanse, be sure to plan ahead and research low-sodium choices. See page 67 for more information on eating out with the Salt Solution in mind.

Q. Should I change my exercise routine during the 2-Week Cleanse?

A. Exercise on the Salt Solution is optional, but physical activity is always helpful if you want to lose weight and improve your health. If you already exercise regularly, by all means keep doing what you're doing. And if you want to start an exercise program or increase your activity levels, we certainly encourage it! Diet and exercise naturally complement each other—like Fred and Ginger or macaroni and cheese. Most experts recommend a minimum of about $2\frac{1}{2}$ hours of exercise per week—or 30 minutes of exercise 5 days a week—but you also can break it into smaller amounts (such as three 10-minute miniworkouts over the course of a day). To help you get moving, check out the Salt Solution Weight-Loss Workout in Chapter 9. It has been specifically designed to help you lose weight while you cut the salt and clean out your diet.

2-Week Cleanse Survival Tips

THERE ARE BOUND TO BE CHALLENGES whenever you start something new, and the Salt Solution Cleanse is no different. We know this phase is restrictive, but with a little forethought, you can learn how to manage challenges and set yourself up for some serious Salt Solution success!

Time It Right: Starting a new job? Moving into a new house? Relocating? The 2-Week Cleanse is not time consuming, but it does require patience and planning, so dealing with the stress of a major life event while starting the Cleanse is not a good idea. Time your Cleanse appropriately so you can concentrate on the weight-loss and sodium-lowering task at hand.

Reduce Temptations: It's just not logical to keep tempting foods around that you know are going to throw you off track. A giant-size bag of salty chips on the kitchen counter, for example, arouses unnecessary temptation. Do yourself a favor and clear your house, office, and car of tempting, unhealthy foods before you start the Cleanse.

Stock Up: Planning your Cleanse meals a week at a time makes grocery shopping a breeze. Fill your kitchen with what you need for the week, and you'll be less likely to stray. Also consider making larger portions of favorite meals to have on hand throughout the week. Some of our test panelists found it helpful to store premade Cleanse meals in individual packages that they could grab on their way out the door. Although it's best to stick to the meals provided in the 2-Week Mix & Match Meals plan, in a pinch you can select from the list of 4-Week Ready-Made Meal Ideas on pages 87–89. Keep a stash of these snacks and meals in your purse, freezer, gym bag, office, and car in case of a missed meal emergency.

Prepare to Eat Out: Again, for optimum results, it's best to eat the Cleanse meals as often as possible, but if dining out is unavoidable during the 2 weeks, try to find out ahead of time where you will be dining. Then look online for a menu and nutrition facts (or call the restaurant to have a menu faxed), and based on the information on pages 217–221, select better-for-you options before you get to the restaurant.

Use Your Food Journal: As we mentioned earlier, documenting why you eat, when you eat, and how much you eat is a powerful tool that can keep you in control—and keep you honest! Filling out a daily food journal will help you make sure excess calories aren't sneaking their way into your diet. (See page 347 to learn how to fill out the food journal.)

Practice Damage Control: If you have an indulgent meal or day, don't let it start a downward spiral. If you get back on the Cleanse with the very next meal and increase your level of activity for a few days, you'll neutralize the impending damage. Many of the test panelists reported that dropping their all-or-nothing attitudes while following the Cleanse not only helped to take the pressure off but also reduced binge eating and increased their focus.

As you reach the end of the 2-Week Cleanse, you'll be feeling energized, lighter, and better than you've felt in years. Your taste buds will be reset and your mineral levels will be restored. You'll also be bloat free and primed for moving on to the next phase of the Salt Solution: the 4-Week Shake the Salt Meal Plan. This phase will provide you with the tools you need to lose the salt and the weight—for life!

Weighing In

Weekly (not daily!) weigh-ins provide a better gauge of where you are in the pounds department. Just be sure to weigh yourself at the same time (preferably in the morning), on the same day of the week, and on the same scale. For best results, weigh yourself in the buff. Note that the scale is not the only way to measure progress. Take body measurements with a tape measure, compare personal photos over time, and assess the fit of your clothing to monitor your improvements.

The Salt Solution
Mineral Boost Juice Options

Please note that each of these makes 1 serving.

Almond, Blueberry, and Banana Smoothie

Combine 1½ cups unsweetened almond milk, ¾ medium frozen banana, 1 cup frozen or fresh blueberries, 1 cup chopped kale, 5 unsalted whole almonds, and 2 teaspoons honey in a blender. Puree until smooth, about 1 to 2 minutes.

Calories: 323
Saturated Fat: 0 g
Fiber: 11 g
Sodium: 300 mg
Potassium: 957 mg
Calcium: 413 mg
Magnesium: 89 mg

Banana-Spinach Smoothie

Combine 1 medium frozen banana, 1 cup fresh spinach, 1 cup plain unsweetened soymilk, 2½ teaspoons almond butter, and 1 teaspoon honey in a blender. Puree until smooth, about 1 to 2 minutes.

Calories: 319
Saturated Fat: 1 g
Fiber: 5 g
Sodium: 174 mg
Potassium: 805 mg
Calcium: 359 mg
Magnesium: 72 mg

Berry-Mango Smoothie

Combine 1 cup chopped kale, ¾ cup frozen mixed berries, ¾ cup fat-free milk, ½ medium frozen banana, ½ cup fresh or frozen mango cubes, and 2 teaspoons honey in a blender. Puree until smooth, about 1 to 2 minutes.

Calories: 321
Saturated Fat: 1 g
Fiber: 4 g
Sodium: 191 mg
Potassium: 934 mg
Calcium: 526 mg
Magnesium: 88 mg

The Salt Solution
2-Week Cleanse Mix & Match Meals

BREAKFASTS

Yogurt Parfait with Berries

Layer 1 cup plain fat-free yogurt with
1 cup sliced strawberries and/or raspberries and 2 tablespoons roasted
unsalted walnuts.

Per serving: 282 calories, 9 g fat, 1 g
saturated fat, 17 g protein, 33 g carbohydrates, 4 g fiber, 191 mg sodium

Cranberries-on-a-Banana

On a medium peeled banana, spread
1 tablespoon all-natural unsalted peanut
butter. Sprinkle with 2 tablespoons dried
cranberries.

Per serving: 289 calories, 13 g fat, 3 g
saturated fat, 7 g protein, 43 g carbohydrates, 5 g fiber, 6 mg sodium

Spinach Scramble

Sauté 2 cups spinach leaves in a nonstick
skillet until wilted. Scramble with 1 egg.
Serve on top of 1 slice whole wheat
bread, toasted. Enjoy with a broiled
brown sugar grapefruit (slice a grapefruit
in half, sprinkle 1 teaspoon brown sugar
over each half, and broil until the sugar
bubbles).

Per serving: 280 calories, 6 g fat, 2 g
saturated fat, 13 g protein, 45 g carbohydrates, 6 g fiber, 257 mg sodium

Hot Couscous Bowl

Combine ½ cup fat-free milk with ¾ cup
cooked couscous. Heat for a minute in
the microwave. Top with 1 cup blueberries and 1 tablespoon chopped pecans.

Per serving: 304 calories, 6 g fat, 1 g
saturated fat, 10 g protein, 56 g carbohydrates, 6 g fiber, 276 mg sodium

Soy Oatmeal

Cook ½ cup rolled oats according to
package directions, using ¾ cup soymilk
instead of milk or water. Top with ½ small
banana, sliced, and 1 teaspoon brown
sugar.

Per serving: 299 calories, 6 g fat, 1 g
saturated fat, 11 g protein, 53 g carbohydrates, 6 g fiber, 92 mg sodium

LUNCHES AND DINNERS

Cinnamon Sweet Potato

Sprinkle 1 small baked sweet potato with
$1/4$ cup dried cranberries, $1/2$ teaspoon
cinnamon, $1/4$ teaspoon cayenne pepper
(optional), and $1/4$ cup plain fat-free
yogurt. Serve with 1 cup steamed
broccoli florets and 1 large apple.

Per serving: 307 calories, 1 g fat, 0 g
saturated fat, 7 g protein, 74 g carbohydrates, 11 g fiber, 289 mg sodium

Sardine Salad

Add 1 teaspoon chopped parsley,
1 teaspoon lemon juice, and 1 small
tomato, chopped, to 1 ounce cooked
sardines (low-sodium canned sardines
are okay). Serve on top of 2 cups spinach
leaves. Dress salad with 1 tablespoon
olive oil and $1 1/2$ tablespoons toasted
pine nuts.

Per serving: 293 calories, 26 g fat, 3 g
saturated fat, 11 g protein, 7 g carbohydrates, 4 g fiber, 196 mg sodium

Fish Taco

Cook 3 ounces halibut in a nonstick pan.
Just before the fish is cooked through,
add 1 cup cooked corn kernels and 1 cup
cherry tomatoes, sliced in quarters.
Serve with 1 small corn tortilla and 1 cup
sliced jicama.

Per serving: 309 calories, 4 g fat, 1 g
saturated fat, 24 g protein, 51 g carbohydrates, 13 g fiber, 110 mg sodium

Edamame Salad

Combine $1/2$ cup cooked edamame with
$1/2$ cup cubed tofu, 1 small tomato,
chopped, 2 teaspoons chopped cilantro,
and 2 teaspoons lemon juice. Drizzle with
1 teaspoon peanut oil.

Per serving: 283 calories, 17 g fat, 3 g
saturated fat, 24 g protein, 15 g carbohydrates, 7 g fiber, 223 mg sodium

Tarragon Chicken Salad

Cube 2 ounces cooked chicken breast.
Toss with 1 tablespoon chopped pecans,
1 teaspoon fresh tarragon, 1 teaspoon
lemon juice, and 1 teaspoon olive oil.
Serve over 2 cups spinach leaves.
Enjoy with 1 cup mango slices.

Per serving: 296 calories, 12 g fat, 2 g
saturated fat, 20 g protein, 31 g carbohydrates, 5 g fiber, 273 mg sodium

Steamed Salmon

Steam 3 ounces salmon. Top with sauce
made from $1/2$ cup fat-free yogurt,
2 teaspoons lemon juice, and 1 teaspoon
fresh dill. Serve on top of 2 cups steamed
spinach. Sprinkle the plate with
1 teaspoon sesame seeds. Enjoy with
1 cup honeydew melon cubes.

Per serving: 286 calories, 7 g fat, 2 g
saturated fat, 29 g protein, 28 g carbohydrates, 3 g fiber, 213 mg sodium

Eggplant Parmesan

Place 2 cups cubed eggplant in a baking dish, top with 2 ounces low-sodium mozzarella cheese, 1 medium tomato, chopped, and 1/2 teaspoon dried oregano. Bake at 375°F for 20 minutes or until tender. Serve with 1 cup beet greens (or spinach) sautéed with 1 clove garlic, minced, until greens are wilted. Enjoy with 1 medium orange.

Per serving: 290 calories, 11 g fat, 6 g saturated fat, 20 g protein, 33 g carbohydrates, 12 g fiber, 104 mg sodium

Pork and Beans

Cook 2 ounces boneless pork loin. Top with 1 small tomato, chopped, 1 teaspoon chopped fresh parsley, and 1 teaspoon lemon juice. Sprinkle with 1/4 cup roasted unsalted soybeans. Serve with 1 cup steamed green beans sprinkled with 2 tablespoons slivered almonds.

Per serving: 285 calories, 14 g fat, 2 g saturated fat, 24 g protein, 18 g carbohydrates, 9 g fiber, 199 mg sodium

Greens and Couscous Salad

In a nonstick pan, sauté 2 cups spinach (or beet greens) with 2 cloves garlic, minced, until greens are wilted. Combine cooked greens with 3/4 cup cooked whole wheat couscous. Top with sauce made from 1/4 cup fat-free yogurt, 1/2 teaspoon cumin, and 1 teaspoon lemon juice. Sprinkle with 2 tablespoons unsalted pine nuts.

Per serving: 301 calories, 12 g fat, 1 g saturated fat, 12 g protein, 38 g carbohydrates, 4 g fiber, 319 mg sodium

Mini Pizza

Top half of a whole wheat English muffin with 1/2 cup chopped tomatoes and 1 ounce low-sodium mozzarella cheese. Serve with a salad made from 2 cups spinach and 1 small carrot, chopped, and dressed with 1 teaspoon olive oil and 2 teaspoons lemon juice. Enjoy with 1 medium orange.

Per serving: 286 calories, 10 g fat, 4 g saturated fat, 15 g protein, 39 g carbohydrates, 9 g fiber, 228 mg sodium

DESSERTS AND SNACKS

No more than one of your three meals per day should be a dessert or snack.

Berry Kebabs

On wooden skewers, arrange the following fruits, cubed: 1 cup strawberries, 1 cup raspberries, and 1 cup blackberries. Dip into a sauce made from ¾ cup low-fat plain yogurt, 1 teaspoon chopped mint, 1 teaspoon brown sugar, and 1 drop vanilla extract.

Per serving: 305 calories, 5 g fat, 2 g saturated fat, 14 g protein, 57 g carbohydrates, 19 g fiber, 134 mg sodium

Chocolate Fondue

Dip 1 small banana (or half of a large banana), sliced, ½ cup cubed honeydew melon, and ½ cup cubed cantaloupe into 1 ounce melted dark chocolate.

Per serving: 295 calories, 10 g fat, 6 g saturated fat, 3 g protein, 55 g carbohydrates, 6 g fiber, 36 mg sodium

PB&J Graham

Spread 1 tablespoon unsalted peanut butter and 1 tablespoon fruit juice–sweetened jam onto 1 graham cracker sheet. Serve with 1 cup fat-free milk.

Per serving: 283 calories, 10 g fat, 2 g saturated fat, 14 g protein, 35 g carbohydrates, 2 g fiber, 195 mg sodium

Orange-Yogurt Pops

Mix ½ cup orange juice with ½ cup fat-free vanilla yogurt. Add a drop of vanilla extract. Freeze in a freezer-pop mold. Enjoy with 25 almonds.

Per serving: 293 calories, 15 g fat, 1 g saturated fat, 14 g protein, 28 g carbohydrates, 4 g fiber, 97 mg sodium

White Bean Hummus

Mash together ½ cup white beans with 1 tablespoon olive oil, 2 teaspoons lemon juice, and ½ teaspoon cumin. Serve with half of a whole wheat pita and 5 baby carrots for dipping.

Per serving: 298 calories, 14 g fat, 2 g saturated fat, 10 g protein, 34 g carbohydrates, 8 g fiber, 317 mg sodium

Salt Solution Success Story

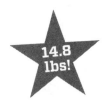

14.8 lbs!

Robin Scholtz

Age: 45

Pounds Lost: 14.8

Inches Lost: 12¼ overall

"I HAVE STRUGGLED WITH MY WEIGHT ALL MY LIFE!" says Robin, a 45-year-old order-entry assistant. Like many dieters, Robin tried (and failed) to drop the pounds with many, many different weight-loss programs. From counting points and counting carbs to detoxing and diet pills, nothing stuck. She would lose a few pounds, but eventually her food cravings would take over, and she would cave and go back to her old eating habits. The missing ingredient in her winning weight-loss recipe? Salt (or *less* salt to be precise).

"For me, salt is an issue. I am what some might call a 'saltaholic.' I would put it on every meal even before I tasted the food. I also ate a lot of prepared and fast foods, which I realize now are sodium laden."

However, with help from the Salt Solution, Robin was able to get her salt addiction under control. This, in turn, helped her drop pounds. "I was astounded at how flavorful foods are *without* all the salt! By offering a variety of healthy, flavorful mini meals using herbs and spices rather than salt, this program helped me control my cravings and change my lifestyle. And by sticking to the initial 'cleansing' phase, I was able to break my salt habit and clear my system of all the toxins, including the excess sodium. This made sticking to the plan and changing my lifestyle so much easier."

Robin wanted this plan to help her turn her life around, and that's exactly what it did. In just 6 weeks, Robin lost almost 15 pounds (more than 10 of them in the first 2 weeks alone!) and more than 12 inches overall. "On the Salt Solution, I have learned how to eat healthier overall. I eat more frequently, and I eat whole foods rather than prepared foods. I love that I can basically eat five times a day and still lose weight and feel good! I've lost a good sum of weight and inches, learned how to eat properly, and I'm taking care of *me* for a change!"

SALT SOLUTION MAKEOVER

Robin's "**Before**" Diet

- **BREAKFAST:** 1 cup canned corned beef hash with 2 slices of wheat toast with 2 tablespoons of butter
- **LUNCH:** Burger King Whopper with a medium fries and soda
- **DINNER:** half of a takeout medium cheese pizza (around 4 slices) and 2 cups of soda
- **SNACK:** 1 bag of buttered microwave popcorn

Robin's "**After**" Diet

- **BREAKFAST:** Egg, Arugula, and Tomato Sandwich (with low-fat Swiss cheese)
- **SNACK:** Berry-Mango Smoothie Mineral Boost Juice
- **LUNCH:** Turkey Burgers with Tomato Relish (with kale)
- **DINNER:** Cilantro-Chicken Stir-Fry (with quinoa, sweet potato, peppers, and peas)
- **SNACK:** Yogurt Parfait with Berries

"**Before**" Nutrition

- **Calories:** 3,935
- **Sodium:** 6,211 mg
- **Saturated Fat:** 81 g
- **Fiber:** 25 g

"**After**" Nutrition

- **Calories:** 1,447
- **Sodium:** 1,224 mg
- **Saturated Fat:** 7 g
- **Fiber:** 31 g

Salt Solution Improvements: Robin not only dramatically decreased her sodium intake (from 6,211 mg to 1,224 mg) and her calories (from 3,935 to 1,447), she also drastically increased her nutrient intake. Robin's diet prior to the Salt Solution was loaded with processed and fast foods like pizza and Whoppers but was seriously lacking in nutrient-rich produce, low-fat dairy, whole grains, and lean protein. By trading large portions of junk foods for small meals filled with healthy ingredients like lean chicken, nuts, yogurt, quinoa, and plenty of fruits and veggies, Robin considerably upped her vitamins, minerals, antioxidants, and fiber. This helped Robin stay satisfied and control her cravings.

THE
4-WEEK
Shake
THE SALT
MEAL PLAN

At this point, you've lost a few pounds, rid yourself of excess sodium, and reset your taste buds. Now, with more confidence and more energy, you're ready to start the 4-Week Shake the Salt Meal Plan. If you've completed the 2-Week Cleanse, this next phase will be a snap! You get more calories, tons of additional meals and recipes to choose from, and tons of flexibility.

The Goals of the 4-Week Shake the Salt Meal Plan

WHY DO YOU WANT TO ADD *more* calories to your diet at this point? The Cleanse lasts just 2 weeks because your metabolism will slow down (as will your weight loss) if you stay on such a low-calorie diet for longer than 2 weeks. In fact, one of the best ways to sabotage weight loss is by eating too little. At first, this seems counterintuitive. You want to lose weight, so you eat less, right? Well, to a point. But once you start eating too little (the exact calorie amount varies from person to person), your body goes into "starvation mode" and starts conserving calories that it needs to perform your basic body functions. This is why it's so important to follow the Salt Solution program meals. Don't be tempted to skip meals in order to save calories! You'll just make it harder to lose weight.

By using the 2-week 1,200-calorie Cleanse to jump-start weight loss and then switching to the 4-week 1,500-calorie Meal Plan, you will keep your metabolism on track and

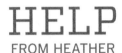

HELP
FROM HEATHER

What if I'm still hungry?

If you find that you're still hungry after eating your Salt Solution meals, try adding some of the foods on the Salt Solution Freebies list (see page 64). It includes nutrient-dense, low-calorie foods you can use to add bulk to your meals without adding many calories.

Before you start increasing your intake, though, be sure your appetite is "real" hunger (hunger of the body), as opposed to "phony" hunger (hunger in the mind). (See Chapter 8 for more on emotional eating.) Phony hunger tends to come on fast and accompanies a gnawing feeling of urgency as well as a craving for something specific—like brownies or cheese puffs. Real hunger, on the other hand, comes on slowly, accompanies a growling stomach, and can be satisfied with lots of foods.

set yourself up for consistent weight loss. And you can keep repeating the 4-Week Shake the Salt Meal Plan for months, or even a year, until you reach your goal.

You will lose about 1 to 2 pounds a week on the Shake the Salt Meal Plan. However, if the scale won't budge, examine your diet and ask yourself if you are really sticking to the plan. Continuing to keep a food journal will help keep you honest about your intake and will help you tackle emotional eating issues (see page 221). If you are actually following the plan and still not dropping pounds, try exercise. If you are already working out, pick it up a notch. If you have yet to lace up those sneakers and get moving, now would be a good time to start. The Salt Solution Weight-Loss Workout in Chapter 9 has been specifically designed to help you lose weight while you reduce sodium.

During the 4-Week Shake the Salt Meal Plan, you will:

Keep On Losing: With your metabolism in check and your salt addiction broken, you'll continue to drop pounds. You can expect to lose about 1 to 2 pounds per week!

Expand Your Palate: Without the taste of salt masking the true flavors of foods and with your taste buds reset, you'll begin to appreciate natural subtle flavors. You'll also experiment with new foods, recipes, and meals to broaden your culinary repertoire. With all these new flavors, you won't want to go back to your old salt-packed ways.

Increase Nutrients: As you continue to eat healthy, clean, low-salt foods, you'll fill your body with the nutrients it needs, especially the Miracle Minerals: potassium, magnesium, and calcium.

Build a Healthy Lifestyle: This plan will teach you how to build healthy habits—for life. The Salt Solution isn't a quick fix. It's meant to be a long-term eating plan so you can remain lean and low-salt for the rest of your life.

4-Week Shake the Salt Meal Plan Basics

D URING THE 4-WEEK SHAKE THE SALT MEAL PLAN, you will eat four 300-calorie meals per day plus drink a daily Mineral Boost Juice. Again, be sure to eat a meal or have a Mineral Boost Juice once every 4 to 5 hours. Your body needs frequent refueling, just like a car, and eating regularly helps prevent extreme hunger and the overeating that often goes with it.

Misunderstood Metabolism

You've heard it before: "I can't lose weight. I have a slow metabolism." What does this mean? And is it even true? Basically, metabolism is the process your body uses to turn food into energy. Your metabolism works to provide you with fuel for exercise, but also energizes your body to perform functions you can't see, like keeping your heart beating and your lungs breathing air. The number of calories needed to perform these hidden functions is your basal metabolic rate. Between 60 and 75 percent of the calories you burn every day are from these hidden body functions.

In addition to the basal metabolic rate, there are two other factors that determine how many calories you burn in a day. One is the digesting, transporting, and processing of the food you eat, also known as *thermogenesis*. Thermogenesis accounts for about 10 percent of the calories you burn in a day. The other is physical activity, which accounts for about 15 to 30 percent of your daily calorie burn.

It's true that some people have a higher basal metabolic rate (that is, a faster metabolism) than others—bigger bodies burn more calories than smaller bodies, men burn more calories than women, and younger people burn more calories than older people. But a slightly lower basal metabolic rate does not mean you can't lose weight. If you eat fewer calories than your body needs, you will lose weight. Period.

Mix & Match Meals and Recipes: Have Four per Day

The 4-Week Shake the Salt Meal Plan is a mix & match meal plan. You will eat four 300-calorie meals per day, and each meal will have approximately 300 milligrams of sodium.

During this phase, you can choose any recipes in this book, including meals from the 2-Week Cleanse, to provide you with your four daily Salt Solution meals. They all have the right number of calories and sodium. (Dessert and sweets recipes and meals should be limited to no more than one per day as they don't provide the same balanced nutrition as the other meals.)

Since all the recipes and the Cleanse meals provide about 300 calories, you can move them around or swap them out at will. For example, a breakfast meal can be eaten for dinner; a snack can be eaten as breakfast, or a lunch meal as a snack. Again, you may repeat meals that you find most enjoyable if you wish, but variety is strongly encouraged. In a pinch you can select from the list of 4-Week Ready-Made Meal Ideas on page 87, but no more than once or twice a week as they are higher in sodium and lower in nutrients than the Salt Solution meals.

Mineral Boost Juice: Have One per Day

As in the 2-Week Cleanse, you will continue to have one daily Mineral Boost Juice, a smoothie pumped with calcium, magnesium, and potassium, the minerals depleted by excess sodium. Again, you can choose from the three versions of the Mineral Boost Juice. Mix and match them any way you please. See page 69 for recipes.

4-WEEK MEAL PLAN Q & A'S

Here are some questions that were frequently asked by our test panelists. Knowing the answers ahead of time will help you achieve optimal success during the 4-Week Shake the Salt Meal Plan.

Q. Can I eat the same meals every day?

A. If you find a few favorite meals you really like, by all means feel free to repeat them as many times as you like. For the best balance in nutrition, though (and to stave off boredom), we encourage you to choose a variety of meals with different foods and try to have fish at least twice a week as recommended by the American Heart Association. However, if you want to have the same Mineral Boost Juice every day, that's fine.

Q. Can I swap out ingredients in a meal or recipe?

A. Yes! While we asked you not to swap out ingredients in a meal during the 2-Week Cleanse, during this phase, you can swap out foods within a meal as long as you substitute like foods for like foods within the building blocks. Swap lean protein for lean protein, a fruit for a fruit, a grain for a grain, almonds for walnuts, etc. Just be sure you're making equivalent calorie swaps. You can check out the USDA nutrient database to get information on calories for different foods at www.nal.usda.gov/fnic/foodcomp/search/.

Q. Do I have to stick to meals from the book?

A. The first time you do the 4-Week Shake the Salt Meal Plan, it's probably best to stick with the meals and recipes in this book, which have been carefully designed to give you the right balance of nutrients. They are low in sodium; high in calcium, magnesium, and potassium; and have just the right balance of protein, carbs, and fats—not to mention they're delicious! Then, once you've become accustomed to eating the Salt Solution way, use the nutrition guidelines listed on page 84 to start creating your own mouthwatering low-sodium dishes.

Q. What if I'm lactose intolerant?

A. Soymilk, soy yogurt, and soy cheese make excellent substitutions for dairy foods. The soybean is the only common plant food that contains "complete" protein, meaning it provides all the essential amino acids needed for human health. And calcium-fortified soy "dairy" products have nutrient levels similar to cow's milk products. Furthermore, soymilk and soybeans are both mineral-rich Salt Solution Stars.

Q. Do I still need to measure my food?

A. We know that it's tiresome to have to measure every time you prepare a meal. But, as we mentioned in the 2-Week Cleanse, it's very easy to overestimate a serving size. For this reason, we recommend that you do continue to measure your food throughout the 4-Week Shake the Salt Meal Plan. Remember, for cup and spoon measurements (1/2 cup, 1 tablespoon, etc.), be sure to level the top.

Q. Can I have coffee, alcohol, and other beverages in this phase?

A. You'll lose weight and inches faster if you stick with the calorie- and carbonation-free choices you've been drinking on the Cleanse: plain water and unsweetened brewed hot and cold green, red, white, black, or herbal tea. During the 4-Week Shake the Salt Meal Plan, though, if you want to add some other beverages for variety, feel free to do so. Just be careful to account for the added calories.

Q. When buying packaged foods, are there any specific foods I should look for at the market?

A. Yes. We recommend looking for brands that are low in sodium (aim for foods that have less than 5 percent of the daily value for sodium) and foods that have 1.5 grams or less of saturated fat per serving, contain no trans fats, are minimally processed, and are free from artificial sweeteners, colors, flavors, preservatives, and high fructose corn syrup. For lots of Salt Solution–approved brands, check out Chapter 7.

Q. Do I have to buy the brands listed in the meal plans?

A. We've selected particular brands because of their taste, quality, availability, sodium level, and nutritional value. Including these foods guarantees steady weight loss because their precise number of calories (and carbohydrate/fiber level) per serving has been incorporated into the plan. We encourage you to use these brands. However, if you can't or prefer not to, simply replace them with comparable foods with as close to the same calorie, sodium, and fiber levels as possible.

Q. Should I exercise during this phase?

A. Although exercise is still optional during this phase, we strongly encourage it. The Salt Solution test panelists who exercised collectively reported that their energy levels soared. Some successfully started an exercise program while on the Salt Solution, and others, who had already been exercising prior to starting the program, found that the plan better fueled their workouts and increased their endurance. The Salt Solution walking program (see page 237) is designed to turn your body into a higher calorie- and fat-burning machine, and the Salt Solution strength-training routine (see page 254) will help you develop even more muscle so you can work off even more calories.

Be Your Own Dietitian

UILDING YOUR OWN SALT SOLUTION MEALS is easy. Using the Salt Solution building blocks listed below, you don't even have to count calories. Just use the serving sizes within the various food groups (protein, dairy, produce, grains, and fat) to build your breakfasts, lunches, dinners, desserts, or snacks. It's easy! All the Salt Solution meals are structured the exact same way. Each has:

One serving of protein

One serving of dairy

One serving of produce

One serving of grains

One serving of fat

Remember that your target is 300—no more than about 300 calories and 300 milligrams of sodium per meal. You'll also want to keep the filling fiber in your meals high (at least 5 grams) and the heart-harming bad fats in your diet low (no more than

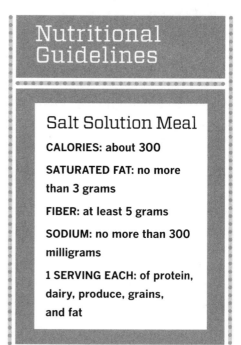

Nutritional Guidelines

Salt Solution Meal

CALORIES: about 300

SATURATED FAT: no more than 3 grams

FIBER: at least 5 grams

SODIUM: no more than 300 milligrams

1 SERVING EACH: of protein, dairy, produce, grains, and fat

3 grams). Stick with the foods listed here and you'll be all set. And be sure to include the Salt Solution Stars and/or the foods listed in Appendix: Where to Find the Miracle Minerals, on page 286, as often as possible.

Keep in mind that it's best to try this only after you've carefully followed the 2-Week Cleanse and the 4-Week Shake the Salt Meal Plan for a few weeks. By creating those meals and recipes, you'll learn about portions and meal components, and this will make it easier for you to build your own Salt Solution meals.

The Salt Solution Meal Building Blocks

To put together your own Salt Solution meal, choose one food from each of the following categories:

Protein (a serving is about 75 calories)

1 to 3 ounces lean meat, poultry, or fish; $\frac{1}{3}$ cup tofu; $\frac{1}{3}$ cup cooked beans or lentils; 1 egg; $\frac{1}{3}$ cup 1% or 2% low-sodium cottage cheese; $1\frac{1}{2}$ ounces reduced-fat hard or semihard cheese; 1 ounce regular cheese*; or 1 tablespoon peanut butter*

*If you have this higher-fat choice, then you have used up a fat serving, too.

Dairy (a serving is about 50 calories)

$\frac{1}{2}$ cup fat-free or 1% milk; $\frac{1}{4}$ cup low-fat or fat-free plain yogurt; $\frac{1}{2}$ cup calcium-enriched soymilk; 1 ounce reduced-fat hard or semihard cheese; or $\frac{1}{2}$ ounce regular cheese*

*If you have this higher-fat choice, then you have used up a fat serving, too.

Produce (a serving is about 50 calories)

Have 2 fruit and 3 vegetable servings daily.

Fruit: a medium-size fruit or 1 cup chopped fruit or berries; $\frac{1}{2}$ cup grapes; 2 tablespoons dried fruit; or $\frac{1}{2}$ cup fruit juice. You can choose any fruit, but be sure to include apples, apricots, bananas, dates, grapefruit, grapefruit juice, grapes, mangoes, melons, oranges, peaches, pineapples, raisins, strawberries, and tangerines.

OR

Vegetables: 2 cups raw leafy vegetables; 1 cup chopped nonleafy vegetables; or 1 cup cooked vegetables. You can choose any vegetable, but be sure to include beet greens, broccoli, carrots, collards, cucumber, green beans, green peas, kale, lima beans, potatoes, spinach, squash, sweet potatoes, and tomatoes.

Grains (a serving is about 75 calories)

½ cup brown rice, whole wheat pasta, or hot whole grain cereal; about 1 cup cold whole grain cereal; 1 slice whole grain bread; one 6" tortilla; or ½ medium bagel or English muffin

Fat (a serving is about 50 calories)

1 teaspoon olive or canola oil; 3 tablespoons chopped avocado; 1 tablespoon nuts; 1 tablespoon ground flaxseed; 2 teaspoons peanut or other nut butter or tahini; or 8 olives

Sample Meal 1: Open-Faced Breakfast Sandwich

Scramble 1 egg in 1 teaspoon olive oil. Toast 1 slice of whole grain bread and top with 1 ounce reduced-fat, low-sodium cheese and the scrambled egg. Enjoy with 1 medium apple.

Sample Meal 2: Mediterranean Chicken Salad

In a bowl, mix ½ cup brown rice, 3 ounces chopped grilled chicken, ½ cup chopped tomatoes, 1 cup spinach leaves, and 8 sliced olives. Combine ¼ cup fat-free plain Greek-style yogurt, 2 teaspoons lemon juice, and 1 tablespoon fresh chopped basil. Fold dressing into rice salad.

Sample Meal 3: Bean Burrito

Wrap ⅓ cup black beans, 1 ounce shredded reduced-fat Cheddar cheese, and 3 tablespoons chopped avocado in a 6" tortilla. Microwave until warm. Serve with ½ cup grapes.

4-Week Ready-Made Meal Ideas

ALTHOUGH THE FOLLOWING ARE GOOD in a pinch, you should limit these meals to no more than once or twice a week as they're not as nutritious as the Salt Solution meals.

Bars

Look for bars with no more than 250 calories, 300 milligrams of sodium, 3 grams of saturated fat, and at least 3 grams of fiber. Have a piece of fruit or a serving of vegetables with each bar to make it a Salt Solution meal.

Bar (per bar)	Calories	Sodium (in milligrams)	Saturated Fat (in grams)	Fiber (in grams)
CLIF Apricot	230	125	0.5	5
CLIF Black Cherry Almond	250	110	1.5	5
CLIF Chocolate Brownie	240	150	1.5	5
CLIF Crunchy Peanut Butter	250	230	1	5
KIND Fruit & Nut Delight	170	25	1.5	4
KIND Nut Delight	200	15	2	4
KIND Walnut & Date	150	40	1	3
Lärabar Apple Pie	190	10	1	5
Lärabar Banana Bread	230	0	1	5
Lärabar Chocolate Coconut Chew	240	0	2.5	5
Lärabar Ginger Snap	240	0	1	6
LUNA Chai Tea	190	95	2.5	3
LUNA Lemon Zest	180	115	2	3
LUNA Nutz Over Chocolate	180	190	2	4
LUNA S'mores	180	140	2	3

Frozen Meals

Look for meals with about 300 calories, no more than 400 milligrams of sodium, no more than about 3 grams of saturated fat, and at least 3 grams of fiber.

Frozen Meal (per meal)	Calories	Sodium (in milligrams)	Saturated Fat (in grams)	Fiber (in grams)
Amy's Light in Sodium Beans & Cheese Burrito	330	290	2.5	7
Amy's Light in Sodium Beans & Rice Burrito	320	290	1	8
Amy's Light in Sodium Black Bean Enchilada	320	380	1	3
Amy's Light in Sodium Brown Rice & Vegetables Bowl	260	270	1	5
Amy's Light in Sodium Indian Mattar Paneer	320	390	1.5	6
Amy's Light in Sodium Vegetable Lasagna	290	340	3.5	4
Amy's Light in Sodium Veggie Loaf Whole Meal	290	340	1	10
Celentano Vegetarian Penne with Roasted Vegetables	300	290	1	8
Kashi Black Bean Mango	340	380	1	7
Kashi Mayan Harvest Bake	340	380	1	8
Kashi Sweet & Sour Chicken	320	380	0.5	6

Soups

Look for soups with no more than 200 calories, 300 milligrams of sodium, 3 grams of saturated fat, and at least 2 grams of fiber. Double the serving if the soup is 100 calories or less, and have a piece of fruit or a serving of vegetables with each soup to make it a Salt Solution meal.

Soup (per cup)	Calories	Sodium (in milligrams)	Saturated Fat (in grams)	Fiber (in grams)
Amy's Light in Sodium Organic Butternut Squash Soup	100	290	0	2
Amy's Light in Sodium Organic Lentil Soup	180	290	1	6
Campbell's Low Sodium Chicken with Noodles Soup	160	140	2	2
Health Valley Organic No Salt Added Black Bean Soup	130	25	0	5
Health Valley Organic No Salt Added Potato Leek Soup	100	290	0	3
Imagine Light in Sodium Organic Creamy Garden Tomato Soup	80	300	0	2
Imagine Light in Sodium Organic Creamy Red Bliss Potato & Roasted Garlic Soup	100	220	0	2
Progresso Reduced Sodium Chicken Gumbo Soup	70	35	0.5	2

Salt Solution Success Story

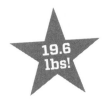

19.6 lbs!

Michael Tonno

Age: 52

Pounds Lost: 19.6

Inches Lost: 6¾ overall

MICHAEL, A 52-YEAR-OLD SALESMAN, gained weight the way many people do. "Once I graduated from college, got married, and started a family, I stopped regular exercise and my weight crept up a few pounds every year." He tried other diets, including cookie and shake meal replacement plans, but none worked over the long term. As soon as he stopped eating the prepared cookies, shakes, or whatever and started eating his normal diet, the weight came back.

Michael says that, before the Salt Solution, he never thought about how much sodium he was eating. While he never added salt to his food, he was eating enormous portions of fast food and processed foods that were packed with sodium. "Probably the most important thing I've realized is that my portion size was way out of control. The sheer volume of food I was consuming was off the charts. Now I am more tuned in to portion size than ever before." For Michael, the biggest surprise with the Salt Solution was how delicious and filling low-sodium food can be. "Now that I eat smaller portions of fresh foods, I really savor and enjoy the taste of the dish. My relationship with food has changed dramatically."

Following the Salt Solution Diet has helped boost Michael's energy levels. "Sometimes I find myself going for a jog at 10:00 p.m.! I'm up to 4 miles now, and I've shaved 15 minutes off my time in the past 4 weeks. I never had the energy to do that before." Another benefit of the Salt Solution? Time shared with his wife, Gretchen, who also completed the plan. They cook and exercise together and enthuse that the plan is "making us an even stronger couple. This year we will be married 27 years!"

SALT SOLUTION MAKEOVER

Michael's "**Before**" Diet

- **BREAKFAST:** Coffee with half-and-half and Splenda, convenience store breakfast sandwich with egg, cheese, and sausage
- **LUNCH:** 2 double cheeseburgers, fries, diet soda
- **SNACK:** Candy bar
- **DINNER:** Pasta with sauce, steak, salad with dressing
- **SNACK:** Ice cream

"**Before**" Nutrition

- **Calories:** 4,401
- **Sodium:** 5,568 mg
- **Saturated Fat:** 102 g
- **Fiber:** 23 g

Michael's "**After**" Diet

- **BREAKFAST:** Coffee with half-and-half, Yogurt Parfait with Berries
- **LUNCH:** Mini Pizza
- **SNACK:** Dried Fruit, Chocolate Chip, Pretzel, and Nut Mix
- **DINNER:** Fish Taco
- **SNACK:** Spinach Hummus with Vegetable Dippers

"**After**" Nutrition

- **Calories:** 1,365
- **Sodium:** 1,033 mg
- **Saturated Fat:** 14 g
- **Fiber:** 47 g

Salt Solution Improvements: It's easy to see why Michael lost 20 pounds in the 6 weeks of the Salt Solution program. He cut his daily calories by more than 3,000 (from 4,401 to 1,365 calories) and slashed his sodium by more than 4,500 mg (from 5,568 mg to 1,033 mg)! Also amazing is that his saturated fat intake dropped from 102 g to 14 g per day. Michael is on his way to a much healthier, fitter life with the Salt Solution.

The Salt

SOLUTION
RECIPES

If you want to decrease the sodium in your diet and enjoy healthy and delicious meals while dropping pounds, eating in is the way to go. Dining at home gives you full control over your choices and your portions and the flexibility to experiment with new flavors and foods. The recipes you'll find here are easy to prepare, and they're so delicious you'll never miss the salt!

Many of these recipes are complete meals as is, but for some you'll need to add a little something to round them out—like a piece of fruit, a quick vegetable side, some bread, or a drink. We've added suggestions in the "Make It a Salt Solution Meal" notes, but feel free to add similar foods within the same food group—a fruit for a fruit, a grain for a grain (such as 1 slice of bread for ½ cup rice), almonds for walnuts, etc. Just be sure you're making equivalent calorie and sodium swaps.

You'll notice that some recipes contain a little more than 300 milligrams of sodium, but don't worry. Since some meals contain less than 300 milligrams of sodium, your daily intake will balance right around 1,200 milligrams of sodium.

In addition to being low in sodium, these meals will give you a healthy dose of your Miracle Minerals. You'll see that many of them incorporate the Salt Solution Stars in creative ways. But these powerhouses aren't the only sources of potassium, calcium, and magnesium, so the recipes include a variety of fruits, vegetables, lean proteins, and other foods rich in these minerals.

BREAKFASTS

Kale and Bell Pepper Omelet

Prep time: 10 minutes · **Cook time:** 11 minutes · **Total time:** 21 minutes · MAKES 1 SERVING

2 large egg whites

1 large egg

2 tablespoons chopped fresh basil

1½ teaspoons canola oil

1½ cups chopped fresh kale

¼ cup water

½ small onion, chopped

½ medium red bell pepper, finely chopped

1 clove garlic, minced

¼ teaspoon dried oregano

1 cup strawberries, hulled and sliced

1. In a medium bowl, whisk together the egg whites, egg, and basil. Set aside.

2. Coat a 10" nonstick skillet with cooking spray. Heat 1 teaspoon of the canola oil in the skillet over medium-high heat. Add the kale and cook until it's just starting to wilt, about 2 minutes. Add the water and cook until it's evaporated, about 3 minutes. Transfer to a plate and reserve. Add the remaining ½ teaspoon oil to the skillet and return to medium-high heat. Add the onion, pepper, garlic, and oregano. Cook, stirring occasionally, until crisp-tender, 4 to 5 minutes. Stir in the kale and cook for 1 minute. Transfer to the plate.

3. Coat the skillet with cooking spray and return to the heat. Pour in the reserved egg mixture and reduce the heat to medium. Cook, lifting the edges to allow the uncooked egg mixture to run underneath, for about 2 minutes, or until the bottom is set. Flip the egg over and cook for 1 minute longer. Top with the kale and onion mixture. Fold half the egg over the filling and slide onto a plate. Serve with the sliced strawberries.

Per serving: 295 calories, 13 g fat, 2 g saturated fat, 19 g protein, 29 g carbohydrates, 7 g fiber, 228 mg sodium

Fruit Omelet

Prep time: 5 minutes ⁑ **Cook time:** 7 minutes ⁑ **Total time:** 12 minutes ⁑ MAKES 2 SERVINGS

    1 cup liquid egg substitute
   ½ cup part-skim ricotta cheese
    1 cup sliced strawberries
      Confectioners' sugar

1. Coat a large skillet with cooking spray and warm over medium heat. When hot, add the egg substitute and cook until almost set.

2. Top half of the egg mixture with the ricotta cheese. Gently fold the other half over the ricotta and continue cooking until the ricotta begins to ooze out of the sides of the omelet.

3. Remove to a large plate and top with the berries. Sprinkle with the sugar.

Per serving: 218 calories, 9 g fat, 4 g saturated fat, 4 g protein, 11 g carbohydrates, 2 g fiber, 300 mg sodium

MAKE IT A SALT SOLUTION MEAL
Serve with 1 small banana (308 calories and 301 mg sodium total).

Egg, Arugula, and Tomato Sandwich

Prep time: 5 minutes ❧ **Cook time:** 3 minutes ❧ **Total time:** 8 minutes ❧ MAKES 1 SERVING

1 light multigrain 100-calorie
    English muffin, split horizontally
1 large egg
1 slice 25% less fat, 53% less
    sodium Swiss cheese

1 tomato slice
¼ cup baby arugula
2 teaspoons unsalted ketchup

1. Toast the English muffin.

2. Meanwhile, coat a small nonstick skillet with cooking spray and heat over medium-high heat. Add the egg, breaking the yolk, and cook for 2 minutes. Turn the egg, top with the cheese, cover, and cook for 1 minute longer, or until the cheese melts and the egg is cooked through. Set the bottom half of the muffin on a plate and top with the tomato slice, arugula, and egg. Spread the cut side of the remaining muffin half with the ketchup and set over the egg. Serve immediately.

Per serving: 207 calories, 8 g fat, 3 g saturated fat, 14 g protein, 28 g carbohydrates, 8 g fiber, 275 mg sodium

Swiss and Turkey Bacon Stratas

Prep time: 25 minutes ⁘ **Cook time:** 45 minutes ⁘ **Total time:** 1 hour 30 minutes ⁘ MAKES 4 SERVINGS

1 small red onion, chopped

½ green bell pepper, chopped

½ red bell pepper, chopped

2 slices extra-lean turkey bacon, chopped (cut crosswise into ¼"-wide strips)

4 slices multigrain bread (4 ounces), cut into ½" cubes

⅓ cup shredded reduced-fat Swiss cheese

2 large eggs

2 large egg whites

1¾ cups 1% milk

1 teaspoon dry mustard

¼ teaspoon freshly ground black pepper

1. Coat a nonstick skillet with cooking spray and heat over medium heat. Add the onion and bell peppers. Cook, stirring occasionally, for 8 minutes, or until the vegetables are almost tender. Stir in the bacon and cook for 2 minutes longer. Remove from the heat and stir in the bread cubes.

2. Coat a 7" × 11" baking dish or four 2-cup casserole dishes with cooking spray and set on a baking sheet. Spoon the vegetable mixture into the baking dish or casserole cups, dividing evenly. Sprinkle on the cheese, dividing evenly.

3. In a medium bowl, whisk together the eggs, egg whites, milk, mustard, and black pepper. Ladle into the baking dish or casserole cups, dividing evenly. Let stand for at least 20 minutes, or cover and refrigerate for up to 12 hours.

4. Preheat the oven to 375°F. Bake the stratas for 35 minutes, or until a knife inserted in the center comes out clean. Let stand for 10 minutes and serve hot.

Per serving: 225 calories, 7 g fat, 3 g saturated fat, 18 g protein, 27 g carbohydrates, 6 g fiber, 316 mg sodium

MAKE IT A SALT SOLUTION MEAL
Serve with 1½ cups watermelon (293 calories and 318 mg sodium total).

Berry-Banana-Ricotta Breakfast Bruschetta

Prep time: 10 minutes ⊳ **Cook time:** 4 minutes ⊳ **Total time:** 14 minutes ⊳ MAKES 4 SERVINGS

1 large banana, sliced
$\frac{1}{2}$ cup sliced fresh strawberries
$\frac{1}{2}$ cup fresh raspberries
2 teaspoons fresh lemon juice
1 teaspoon sugar

$\frac{3}{4}$ cup part-skim ricotta cheese
5 teaspoons honey
4 tablespoons sliced almonds
8 slices raisin bread, toasted

1. In a medium bowl, combine the banana, strawberries, raspberries, lemon juice, and sugar. In a small bowl, combine the ricotta and honey.

2. Heat a small nonstick skillet over medium heat. Add the almonds and cook, shaking the skillet occasionally, until they are lightly toasted, about 4 minutes. Transfer to a bowl and cool.

3. Spread 1 side of each toast slice with the ricotta mixture. Place 2 slices onto each of 4 serving plates. Top each with one-eighth of the banana mixture. Sprinkle each with $\frac{1}{2}$ tablespoon of the almonds and serve immediately.

Per serving: 325 calories, 9 g fat, 3 g saturated fat, 11 g protein, 53 g carbohydrates, 6 g fiber, 262 mg sodium

French Toast with Banana-Berry Topping

Prep time: 10 minutes ⋮· **Cook time:** 10 minutes ⋮· **Total time:** 20 minutes ⋮· MAKES 4 SERVINGS

1 teaspoon unsalted butter
3 medium bananas, sliced
1 cup sliced strawberries
½ cup blueberries
1 tablespoon maple syrup
3 large eggs

1 large egg white
¼ cup fat-free milk
½ teaspoon vanilla extract
⅛ teaspoon ground cinnamon
4 slices multigrain bread

1. Melt the butter in a medium nonstick skillet over medium-high heat. Add the bananas, strawberries, blueberries, and maple syrup. Cook, stirring occasionally, until the fruit is softened, about 4 minutes. Keep warm.

2. In a large bowl, beat together the eggs, egg white, milk, vanilla extract, and cinnamon. Coat a large nonstick skillet with cooking spray and heat over medium-high heat. Working 1 slice at a time, dip both sides of the bread into the egg mixture to coat. Add to the hot skillet and cook until lightly browned, about 3 minutes per side. Place 1 slice onto each of 4 plates, and spoon one-quarter of the fruit mixture over each and serve.

Per serving: 314 calories, 7 g fat, 2 g saturated fat, 14 g protein, 53 g carbohydrates, 10 g fiber, 286 mg sodium

Sweet Potato Pancakes

Prep time: 20 minutes ⁝⊳ **Cook time:** 20 minutes ⁝⊳ **Total time:** 40 minutes ⁝⊳ MAKES 4 SERVINGS

2 sweet potatoes (1¼ pounds), peeled and shredded

1 large tart cooking apple (8 ounces), peeled, cored, and shredded

2 scallions, chopped

2 tablespoons chopped fresh dill

3 tablespoons whole grain pastry flour

¼ teaspoon salt

2 egg whites

1½ teaspoons olive oil

¼ cup unsweetened applesauce

2 tablespoons reduced-fat sour cream

1. In a large bowl, stir together the potatoes, apple, scallions, dill, flour, salt, and egg whites.

2. Preheat the oven to 300°F. Coat a 10" skillet with cooking spray and heat over medium-low heat. Add ¾ teaspoon of the oil and swirl in the pan to coat.

3. For each pancake, drop ½ cup of the sweet potato mixture into the skillet, making 4 pancakes at a time, flattening each with a spatula to a 4" round. Cook for 10 minutes, or until golden brown, turning with a spatula halfway through the cooking time.

4. Place on a baking sheet and keep warm in the oven. Repeat with the remaining ¾ teaspoon oil and the remaining sweet potato mixture. Top the pancakes with the applesauce and sour cream.

Per serving: 203 calories, 3 g fat, 1 g saturated fat, 5 g protein, 41 g carbohydrates, 6 g fiber, 255 mg sodium

MAKE IT A SALT SOLUTION MEAL
Serve with ½ cup fat-free milk and ½ cup blueberries (288 calories and 320 mg sodium total).

Banana Oatmeal Pancakes with Berries

Prep time: 10 minutes ⁖ **Cook time:** 7 minutes per batch ⁖ **Total time:** 17 minutes
⁖ MAKES 4 SERVINGS OF 3 PANCAKES AND ½ CUP BERRIES

1 cup quick-cooking oats
⅔ cup all-purpose flour
2 tablespoons sugar
1 teaspoon baking powder
⅛ teaspoon salt
2 large eggs

1 cup fat-free milk
2 medium bananas, halved lengthwise and sliced
1 cup fresh strawberries, hulled
and sliced
1 cup fresh blueberries

1. In a medium bowl, combine the oats, flour, 4 teaspoons of the sugar, baking powder, and salt.

2. In a separate bowl, combine the eggs and milk. Pour the egg mixture into the oat mixture, stirring until just moistened. Gently fold in the bananas with a rubber spatula.

3. Preheat the oven to 225°F. Coat a large nonstick skillet with cooking spray and heat over medium heat. Spoon four ¼-cupfuls of batter into the skillet and cook until the tops begin to bubble slightly, about 3 to 3½ minutes. Turn the pancakes and cook for 3 to 3½ minutes longer, or until golden and cooked through. Transfer to a baking sheet and keep warm in the oven. Repeat with the remaining batter.

4. Meanwhile, in a medium bowl, toss the berries with the remaining 2 teaspoons sugar. Serve the pancakes topped with the berries.

Per serving: 313 calories, 4 g fat, 1 g saturated fat, 12 g protein, 60 g carbohydrates, 5 g fiber, 257 mg sodium

Breakfast in a Muffin

Prep time: 20 minutes ⋮⋗ **Cook time:** 22 minutes ⋮⋗ **Total time:** 42 minutes ⋮⋗ MAKES 12 MUFFINS

1¼ cups finely crushed whole grain wheat cereal, such as Total

¾ cup all-purpose flour

½ cup stone-ground whole wheat flour

2 teaspoons baking powder

1 teaspoon ground cinnamon

½ teaspoon baking soda

½ teaspoon salt

½ teaspoon ground ginger

¼ teaspoon ground nutmeg

1 teaspoon grated orange zest

2 egg whites

3 tablespoons extra virgin olive oil

1 teaspoon vanilla extract

½ cup packed light brown sugar

½ cup fat-free plain Greek-style yogurt

¼ cup orange juice

⅓ cup golden raisins

1¼ cups fresh or frozen blueberries

5½ tablespoons coarsely chopped almonds

1 tablespoon sugar

1. Preheat the oven to 400°F. Line a 12-cup muffin pan with paper liners.

2. In a large bowl, whisk together the cereal, flours, baking powder, cinnamon, baking soda, salt, ginger, nutmeg, and orange zest. In a medium bowl, whisk together the egg whites, oil, and vanilla extract. Whisk in the brown sugar, yogurt, and orange juice just until blended. Stir into the dry ingredients just until blended.

3. Fold in the raisins and blueberries. Spoon into the muffin cups, nearly filling the cups.

4. In a small bowl, stir together the almonds and turbinado sugar. Sprinkle about 1½ teaspoons over each muffin.

5. Bake for 22 minutes, or until the top of a muffin springs back when lightly touched. Cool on a rack in the pan for 2 minutes. Transfer the muffins to the rack and cool completely.

Per serving: 201 calories, 4 g fat, 1 g saturated fat, 4 g protein, 38 g carbohydrates, 2 g fiber, 319 mg sodium

MAKE IT A SALT SOLUTION MEAL
Serve with 1 medium grapefruit (283 calories and 319 mg sodium total).

Fast and Fruity Oatmeal Bowl

Prep time: 5 minutes ⦂ **Cook time:** 2 minutes ⦂ **Total time:** 7 minutes ⦂ MAKES 1 SERVING

   1 packet plain instant oatmeal
$^2/_3$ cup 1% milk
   1 tablespoon low-fat vanilla yogurt
$1^1/_2$ cups sliced strawberries

In a microwaveable bowl, mix the oats and milk. Microwave for 1 to 2 minutes. Top with the yogurt and strawberries.

Per serving: 260 calories, 4 g fat, 1 g saturated fat, 12 g protein, 48 g carbohydrates, 10 g fiber, 163 mg sodium

MAKE IT A SALT SOLUTION MEAL
Serve with 1 tablespoon unsalted walnuts (347 calories and 165 mg sodium total).

Berry Nut Topped Oatmeal

Prep time: 5 minutes ⸭ **Cook time:** 5 minutes ⸭ **Total time:** 10 minutes ⸭ MAKES 1 SERVING

$3/4$ cup fat-free milk

$1/4$ cup water

2 teaspoons honey

$1/8$ teaspoon almond extract

$1/2$ cup rolled oats

$1/3$ cup fresh blueberries

1 tablespoon sliced almonds

In a small saucepan over medium-high heat, combine the milk, water, honey, and almond extract. Bring to a simmer, stir in the oats, and cook, stirring occasionally, for 5 minutes. Transfer to a bowl and top with the blueberries and almonds.

Per serving: 321 calories, 6 g fat, 1 g saturated fat, 14 g protein, 56 g carbohydrates, 6 g fiber, 80 mg sodium

Baked Rice and Raisin Pudding

Prep time: 8 minutes ▷ **Cook time:** 1 hour 15 minutes ▷ **Total time:** 1 hour 53 minutes
▷ MAKES 6 SERVINGS

2 cans (12 ounces each) evaporated
  fat-free milk
3 tablespoons raisins
1 tablespoon ground flaxseed
½ teaspoon cinnamon

1 egg
2 teaspoons vanilla extract
½ cup brown rice
6 teaspoons brown sugar or honey

1. Preheat the oven to 325°F. Lightly coat an 8" × 8" baking dish with canola oil spray. In a small saucepan, heat the milk for about 3 minutes, or until hot but not boiling.

2. In a spice grinder or small food processor fitted with a metal blade, combine the raisins, flaxseed, and cinnamon. Process for about 2 minutes, or until the raisins are finely chopped. Place in the baking dish.

3. In a mixing bowl, beat the egg with a fork. Add about ½ cup of the milk, beating constantly, to warm the egg. Add the remaining milk and the vanilla extract. Stir to mix.

4. Pour into the baking dish. Add the rice. Stir with a fork. Cover with foil. Bake for 1 hour 15 minutes. Turn off the heat. Let stand in the oven for 30 minutes. Serve right away or cool to room temperature before refrigerating. Serve cold or warm garnished with 1 teaspoon brown sugar or honey.

Note: This dish can be made ahead of time.

Per serving: 202 calories, 2 g fat, 0 g saturated fat, 10 g protein, 36 g carbohydrates, 19 g fiber, 157 mg sodium

MAKE IT A SALT SOLUTION MEAL
Serve with 1 cup grapes (306 calories and 160 mg sodium total).

Breakfast Berry "Sundaes"

Prep time: 10 minutes ⁑ **Total time:** 10 minutes ⁑ MAKES 4 SERVINGS

2 cups fat-free plain Greek-style yogurt

$1/2$ teaspoon vanilla extract

2 tablespoons toasted wheat germ

$1/2$ teaspoon ground cinnamon

3 tablespoons dried cranberries or cherries

3 tablespoons granola or muesli

2 cups (1 pint) blueberries

1 medium banana, sliced

$1/2$ cup toasted slivered almonds

Divide the yogurt among 4 bowls, reserving $1/4$ cup. Drizzle the vanilla extract over the yogurt in each bowl and sprinkle with the wheat germ and cinnamon. Scatter the cranberries or cherries and granola or muesli over each. Spoon $1/2$ cup blueberries over each, then top with the banana slices. Top each serving with 1 tablespoon of the remaining yogurt and sprinkle with the almonds.

Per serving: 257 calories, 9 g fat, 1 g saturated fat, 11 g protein, 40 g carbohydrates, 6 g fiber, 71 mg sodium

MAKE IT A SALT SOLUTION MEAL
Serve with 1 hard-cooked or poached egg sprinkled with fresh chopped chives (325 calories and 193 mg sodium total).

Greek Yogurt with Walnuts and Honey

Prep time: 5 minutes ⋙ **Cook time:** 5 minutes ⋙ **Total time:** 10 minutes ⋙ MAKES 1 SERVING

 2 tablespoons walnut halves,
   chopped
 1 cup fat-free plain Greek-style
   yogurt
 4 teaspoons honey
 ¼ cup raspberries

1. Heat a small skillet over medium heat. Add the walnuts and cook, shaking the skillet often, until lightly toasted, about 4 to 5 minutes. Transfer to a bowl and cool for 5 minutes.

2. Spoon the yogurt into a small bowl and top with the cooled walnuts. Drizzle the honey over the top and add in the raspberries. Serve immediately.

Per serving: 320 calories, 9 g fat, 1 g saturated fat, 16 g protein, 47 g carbohydrates, 3 g fiber, 190 mg sodium

Two-Citrus Breakfast Parfait

Prep time: 10 minutes ⸭ MAKES 2 SERVINGS

½ cup fresh pink grapefruit sections
½ cup fresh orange sections
1 medium banana, sliced
1 cup fat-free plain Greek-style yogurt

2 tablespoons agave nectar
1 cup whole grain wheat cereal, such as Total
20 blueberries

1. In a small bowl, combine the grapefruit, orange, and banana.

2. Spoon ¼ cup yogurt into the bottom of each of 2 parfait glasses. Top each with ⅓ cup of the fruit mixture, 1½ teaspoons agave nectar, and ¼ cup cereal. Repeat layering one more time and top each parfait with 10 blueberries. Serve.

Per serving: 286 calories, 1 g fat, 0 g saturated fat, 13 g protein, 61 g carbohydrates, 5 g fiber, 169 mg sodium

LUNCHES

Mini Eggplant Pizzas

Prep time: 12 minutes ⫸· **Cook time:** 13 minutes ⫸· **Total time:** 25 minutes ⫸· MAKES 4

2 eggplants (each 3" diameter), peeled and each cut into 4 slices ½" thick

2 tablespoons olive oil

¼ teaspoon salt

⅛ teaspoon ground black pepper

2 large ripe tomatoes, each cut into 4 slices

¾ teaspoon dried oregano

½ teaspoon dried basil

¾ teaspoon garlic powder

1 cup (2½ ounces) shredded fat-free mozzarella

1. Preheat the oven or toaster oven to 425°F.

2. Brush both sides of the eggplant slices with the oil and season with the salt and pepper. Arrange on a baking sheet and bake until browned and almost tender, 6 to 8 minutes, turning once.

3. Place a tomato slice on each eggplant slice and season with the oregano, basil, and garlic powder. Top with the cheese and bake until the cheese melts, 3 to 5 minutes. Serve hot.

Per serving: 190 calories, 8 g fat, 1 g saturated fat, 13 g protein, 22 g carbohydrates, 11 g fiber, 283 mg sodium

MAKE IT A SALT SOLUTION MEAL
Serve with a salad made from 1 cup spinach, 2 tablespoons cubed avocado, 1 teaspoon olive oil, and 1 teaspoon fresh lemon juice (267 calories and 308 mg sodium total).

Chicken Parmesan Sandwich

Prep time: 15 minutes ⁝⁝ **Cook time:** 15 minutes ⁝⁝ **Total time:** 30 minutes ⁝⁝ MAKES 4 SERVINGS

4 (4-ounce) boneless, skinless chicken breast halves

4 teaspoons extra virgin olive oil

4 cloves garlic, minced

1 teaspoon dried basil

$\frac{1}{2}$ teaspoon dried oregano

$1\frac{1}{2}$ cups unsalted diced tomatoes

2 tablespoons unsalted tomato paste

4 cups fresh spinach

3 ounces Italian bread, cut diagonally into 4 long, thin slices, toasted

4 tablespoons grated Parmesan cheese

1. In a bowl, combine the chicken and 1 teaspoon of the oil. Turn to coat and set aside.

2. Heat 2 teaspoons of the remaining oil in a medium saucepan over medium-high heat. Add half of the garlic, and the basil and oregano. Cook, stirring often, for 30 seconds. Add the tomatoes and tomato paste, reduce the heat to medium, and simmer until thickened, about 10 minutes. Remove from the heat and keep warm.

3. Meanwhile, heat a nonstick grill pan over medium-high heat. Add the reserved chicken and cook, turning once, for 9 to 10 minutes, or until a thermometer inserted into the thickest portion registers 165°F. While the chicken cooks, heat the remaining 1 teaspoon oil in a large nonstick skillet over medium-high heat. Add the remaining garlic and cook until just starting to brown, about 15 seconds. Add the spinach and cook, stirring occasionally, until wilted, about 2 to 3 minutes.

4. Place 1 slice of toast on each of 4 plates. Top each with $\frac{1}{2}$ cup of the spinach, 1 chicken breast half, one-quarter of the tomato sauce, and 1 tablespoon grated cheese. Serve immediately.

Per serving: 274 calories, 9 g fat, 2 g saturated fat, 29 g protein, 17 g carbohydrates, 2 g fiber, 315 mg sodium

Turkey Burgers with Tomato Relish

Prep time: 15 minutes ⋮► **Cook time:** 15 minutes ⋮► **Total time:** 30 minutes ⋮► MAKES 4 SERVINGS

2 medium tomatoes, seeded and chopped

2 tablespoons chopped fresh basil

2 teaspoons balsamic vinegar

1 teaspoon sugar

$\frac{1}{2}$ teaspoon grated orange zest

1 pound ground turkey breast

$\frac{1}{2}$ teaspoon ground cumin

$\frac{1}{2}$ teaspoon dried basil

$\frac{1}{4}$ teaspoon garlic powder

$\frac{1}{4}$ teaspoon ground coriander

1 teaspoon olive oil

3 cups chopped fresh kale

4 light multigrain 100-calorie English muffins, toasted

1. In a small bowl, combine the tomatoes, fresh basil, vinegar, sugar, and orange zest. Set aside.

2. In a medium bowl, combine the turkey breast, cumin, basil, garlic powder, and coriander. Mix well. Divide the turkey mixture into 4 portions and form each into a $3\frac{1}{2}$"-diameter patty. Coat a grill pan with cooking spray and heat over medium-high heat. Add the turkey patties and cook until a thermometer inserted into the thickest portion registers 175°F, about $4\frac{1}{2}$ to 5 minutes per side.

3. Meanwhile, heat the oil in a medium nonstick skillet over medium-high heat. Add the kale and cook, tossing occasionally, until wilted, about 3 to 4 minutes.

4. Set the bottom half of each English muffin on a plate. Top each with $\frac{1}{4}$ cup tomato relish, a turkey burger, one-quarter of the kale, and the top half of each muffin. Serve immediately.

Per serving: 289 calories, 4 g fat, 1 g saturated fat, 33 g protein, 33 g carbohydrates, 10 g fiber, 306 mg sodium

Turkey Spinach Medley on Pita

Prep time: 10 minutes ❧ **Cook time:** 25 minutes ❧ **Total time:** 35 minutes ❧ MAKES 4 SERVINGS

2 teaspoons olive oil
2 cloves garlic, minced
½ medium onion, chopped
12 ounces lean ground turkey breast

1 package (10 ounces) frozen chopped spinach, thawed and squeezed dry
Ground black pepper
4 whole wheat pitas, halved
1 medium tomato, chopped

1. Warm the oil in a large skillet over medium-high heat. When hot, add the garlic and onion and cook for about 5 minutes, or until tender.

2. Add the turkey and cook, breaking up the turkey with the back of a spoon as you stir, for 15 minutes, or until no longer pink. Add the spinach and cook for 5 to 7 minutes longer, or until the spinach is heated through.

3. Season with pepper to taste and spoon equal portions into the pitas. Top with the tomato and serve.

Per serving: 264 calories, 4 g fat, 1 g saturated fat, 27 g protein, 31 g carbohydrates, 6 g fiber, 329 mg sodium

MAKE IT A SALT SOLUTION MEAL
Serve with 1 orange (309 calories and 329 mg sodium total).

Sizzling Beef Kebabs

Prep time: 10 minutes ⁖ **Cook time:** 2 hours 10 minutes ⁖ **Total time:** 2 hours 20 minutes
⁖ MAKES 4 SERVINGS

8 ounces orange juice with added calcium

5 teaspoons reduced-sodium soy sauce

1 tablespoon rice wine vinegar or apple cider vinegar

2 large cloves garlic, minced

1 tablespoon chopped fresh ginger

$\frac{1}{2}$ teaspoon crushed red-pepper flakes

2 teaspoons ground black pepper

1 teaspoon orange zest

1 pound bottom round, trimmed and cut into $1\frac{1}{2}$" cubes

1 large zucchini, sliced $\frac{1}{2}$" thick

1 yellow bell pepper, cut into 2" chunks

1 red bell pepper, cut into 2" chunks

1. In a flat baking dish, whisk together the orange juice, soy sauce, vinegar, garlic, ginger, red-pepper flakes, black pepper, and orange zest. Place the beef, zucchini, and bell peppers in the dish, coating well with the marinade.

2. Cover the dish with plastic wrap. Marinate in the refrigerator for at least 2 hours.

3. Preheat the grill. Alternate the beef and vegetables on eight 8" or four 10" to 12" skewers. Place the kebabs over the heat and grill each side for 4 to 5 minutes, or until cooked through.

Per serving: 215 calories, 6 g fat, 2 g saturated fat, 28 g protein, 15 g carbohydrates, 3 g fiber, 300 mg sodium

MAKE IT A SALT SOLUTION MEAL
Serve with $\frac{1}{2}$ cup cooked brown rice (323 calories and 305 mg sodium total).

Tuna Steak Sandwich with Lemon-Basil Mayo

Prep time: 15 minutes ⋙ **Cook time:** 16 minutes ⋙ **Total time:** 31 minutes ⋙ MAKES 4 SERVINGS

¼ cup reduced-fat mayonnaise

2 tablespoons chopped fresh basil

2 teaspoons fresh lemon juice

1 teaspoon grated lemon zest

1 medium red onion, cut into 4 (¼"-thick) slices

1 tablespoon extra virgin olive oil

¼ teaspoon freshly ground black pepper

4 (4-ounce) tuna steaks (½" thick)

4 slices whole wheat French bread

1 cup fresh spinach or arugula

1 medium tomato, cut into 4 slices

4 fresh basil leaves

1. In a small bowl, combine the mayonnaise, basil, lemon juice, and lemon zest. Set aside.

2. Preheat the grill. Brush the onion slices with 1 teaspoon of the oil and sprinkle with ⅛ teaspoon of the pepper. Place on the grill and cook for 6 to 7 minutes, turning once, until well marked and tender. Remove from the grill and set aside. Brush the tuna with 1 teaspoon of the remaining oil and sprinkle with the remaining ⅛ teaspoon pepper. Place the tuna steaks on the grill and cook for 6 to 7 minutes, turning once, until pink in the middle. Brush the bread slices with the remaining 1 teaspoon oil and grill for 1 minute per side.

3. Set a bread slice on each of 4 plates and spread the tops with 1 tablespoon of the mayonnaise mixture. Top with ¼ cup spinach or arugula. Top each with an onion slice, a tuna steak, and 1 tomato slice. Place 1 basil leaf in the center of each tomato and serve.

Per serving: 233 calories, 3 g fat, 1 g saturated fat, 30 g protein, 20 g carbohydrates, 2 g fiber, 322 mg sodium

MAKE IT A SALT SOLUTION MEAL
Serve with 1 peach (292 calories and 322 mg sodium total).

Halibut Sandwich
with Easy Tartar Sauce

Prep time: 10 minutes **Cook time:** 10 minutes **Total time:** 20 minutes MAKES 4 SERVINGS

2 tablespoons low-sodium reduced-calorie mayonnaise

1 tablespoon sweet pickle relish

1 tablespoon finely chopped onion

4 (4-ounce) skinless halibut fillets

$\frac{1}{4}$ teaspoon ground black pepper

4 whole wheat hamburger buns

1 medium tomato, cut into 4 slices

4 medium lettuce leaves

1. In a small bowl, combine the mayonnaise, relish, and onion. Mix well. Set aside.

2. Coat a nonstick grill pan with cooking spray and heat over medium-high heat. Sprinkle the halibut fillets with the pepper and add to the pan. Cook, turning once, for 9 to 10 minutes, or until the fish flakes easily with a fork. Remove from the heat.

3. Meanwhile, toast the buns and set 1 bottom on each of 4 plates. Top each with 1 tomato slice, 1 lettuce leaf, and 1 halibut fillet. Spread the top half of each bun with the tartar sauce and set onto the fillet.

Per serving: 302 calories, 7 g fat, 1 g saturated fat, 34 g protein, 26 g carbohydrates, 4 g fiber, 324 mg sodium

Tofu-Spinach Wrap

Prep time: 5 minutes ▷ **Cook time:** 7 minutes ▷ **Total time:** 12 minutes ▷ MAKES 1 SERVING

½ teaspoon ground coriander

⅛ teaspoon ground turmeric

⅛ teaspoon crushed red-pepper flakes

⅛ teaspoon ground black pepper

1 tablespoon water

⅓ cup finely chopped drained firm tofu

½ teaspoon canola oil

2 cups loosely packed spinach, coarsely chopped

1 whole wheat tortilla (8" diameter)

1. In a medium bowl, mix the coriander, turmeric, red-pepper flakes, and black pepper with the water. Add the tofu and toss to coat with the spice mixture.

2. Warm the oil in a medium nonstick skillet over medium-high heat. Add the tofu and cook, stirring, for 5 minutes, or until heated and crisp. Add the spinach and cook, stirring, until wilted, about 1 minute.

3. Remove from the heat and warm the tortilla by placing it over the spinach mixture for about a minute. Spoon the mixture onto the tortilla and roll up, folding in the sides.

Per serving: 175 calories, 7 g fat, 1 g saturated fat, 12 g protein, 24 g carbohydrates, 4 g fiber, 225 mg sodium

MAKE IT A SALT SOLUTION MEAL
Serve with 6 ounces fat-free Greek-style yogurt and ½ cup blueberries (307 calories and 290 mg sodium total).

Lemony Chicken Breast over Beet Greens

Prep time: 10 minutes ⁜ **Cook time:** 10 minutes ⁜ **Total time:** 20 minutes + chilling and standing time ⁜ MAKES 4 SERVINGS

4 (4-ounce) boneless, skinless chicken breast halves

1 tablespoon fresh lemon juice

2 cloves garlic, minced

4 teaspoons extra virgin olive oil

$\frac{1}{8}$ teaspoon ground black pepper

3 cloves garlic, sliced

1 medium onion, thinly sliced

8 cups fresh beet greens

$\frac{1}{8}$ teaspoon salt

1. In a bowl, combine the chicken, lemon juice, garlic, 1 teaspoon of the oil, and pepper. Refrigerate for 1 hour.

2. Remove the chicken from the refrigerator and let stand for 15 minutes at room temperature. Heat a nonstick grill pan over medium-high heat. Add the chicken and cook, turning once, for 9 to 10 minutes, or until a thermometer inserted into the thickest portion registers 165°F.

3. While the chicken cooks, heat the remaining 1 tablespoon oil in a large nonstick skillet over medium-high heat. Add the sliced garlic and onion and cook, stirring occasionally, for about 4 to 5 minutes, or until slightly softened and the garlic begins to brown. Add the beet greens and cook, stirring often, until wilted, about 4 minutes. Stir in the salt.

4. To serve, make a bed of the greens on each of 4 plates. Top each with 1 chicken breast half.

Per serving: 196 calories, 7 g fat, 1 g saturated fat, 25 g protein, 8 g carbohydrates, 3 g fiber, 301 mg sodium

 MAKE IT A SALT SOLUTION MEAL
Serve with a salad made from 1 cup arugula, 5 cherry tomatoes, 1 teaspoon olive oil, and 1 teaspoon balsamic vinegar (266 calories and 316 mg sodium total).

Toasted Almond and Chicken Salad

Prep time: 10 minutes ▸ **Cook time:** 10 minutes ▸ **Total time:** 20 minutes + chilling and standing time ▸ MAKES 4 SERVINGS

3 (4-ounce) boneless, skinless chicken breast halves

3 ribs celery, sliced

1 bunch chives, finely chopped

1/2 cup low-fat plain yogurt

1/4 cup light sour cream

1 1/2 teaspoons dried tarragon

2 tablespoons slivered almonds, toasted

1/4 teaspoon salt

1/8 teaspoon ground black pepper

1 bag (10 ounces) mixed greens

1. Coat a nonstick skillet with cooking spray and heat over medium-high.

2. When the skillet is hot, add the chicken and cook for 4 minutes per side, or until a thermometer inserted into the thickest portion registers 165°F. Remove the chicken from the heat and let it rest for at least 10 minutes.

3. When they're cool enough to handle, chop the chicken breasts into small pieces. In a large bowl, combine the chicken, celery, chives, yogurt, sour cream, and tarragon. Mix lightly. Cover and refrigerate for at least 1 hour, or up to 24 hours.

4. Add the almonds, salt, and pepper. Serve on a bed of greens.

Per serving: 175 calories, 5 g fat, 2 g saturated fat, 25 g protein, 8 g carbohydrates, 3 g fiber, 294 mg sodium

MAKE IT A SALT SOLUTION MEAL
For dessert, drizzle 1 tablespoon melted dark chocolate chips over 1/2 cup sliced strawberries (272 calories and 300 mg sodium total).

Roast Turkey, Orange, and Cashew Salad

Prep time: 8 minutes ⁝· **Total time:** 8 minutes ⁝· MAKES 2 SERVINGS

4 cups mixed salad greens

1 cup fresh spinach

6 ounces (1½ cups) chopped cooked skinless turkey breast

1 can (8½ ounces) mandarin orange segments in light syrup, drained

3 tablespoons low-fat honey mustard dressing

1 tablespoon orange marmalade

2 tablespoons chopped cashews

1. In a bowl, toss the salad greens and spinach. Divide between 2 plates.

2. In the same bowl, combine the turkey, orange segments, dressing, marmalade, and cashews and toss well.

3. Spoon the turkey mixture evenly over the greens and serve.

Per serving: 323 calories, 6 g fat, 1 g saturated fat, 29 g protein, 38 g carbohydrates, 4 g fiber, 265 mg sodium

Sicilian Tuna Salad

Prep time: 15 minutes ⬝ **Cook time:** 3 minutes ⬝ **Total time:** 18 minutes ⬝ MAKES 2 SERVINGS

- 1/4 pound green beans, trimmed and halved crosswise
- 6 cups baby spinach
- 1 can (5 ounces) very low-sodium solid white albacore tuna, drained
- 16 grape tomatoes, halved
- 1 cucumber, peeled, halved lengthwise, and sliced
- 1/2 small red onion, thinly sliced (about 1/4 cup)
- 1/2 cup orange segments
- 2 tablespoons fresh lemon juice
- 1 tablespoon extra virgin olive oil
- 1/8 teaspoon salt

1. Bring a medium saucepan of water to a boil over high heat. Add the green beans, return to a boil, and cook until crisp-tender, about 3 minutes. Drain and rinse under cold water, then drain again.

2. Transfer the green beans to a large bowl, then add the spinach, tuna, tomatoes, cucumber, onion, orange segments, lemon juice, olive oil, and salt. Toss well. Divide between 2 plates and serve.

Per serving: 252 calories, 9 g fat, 2 g saturated fat, 19 g protein, 28 g carbohydrates, 9 g fiber, 302 mg sodium

MAKE IT A SALT SOLUTION MEAL
Serve with 1 tablespoon unsalted almonds (304 calories and 303 mg sodium total).

Curried Egg Salad over Spinach

Prep time: 15 minutes ❧ **Cook time:** 15 minutes ❧ **Total time:** 30 minutes ❧ MAKES 4 SERVINGS

6 large eggs
1 can (15 ounces) no-salt-added cannellini beans, rinsed and drained
½ cup chopped celery
½ cup chopped cucumber
⅓ cup dried apricots, chopped

¼ cup chopped red onion
1 cup fat-free plain yogurt
¼ cup reduced-fat mayonnaise
¼ cup chopped fresh cilantro
1 tablespoon fresh lemon juice
2 teaspoons curry powder
6 cups fresh spinach

1. Put the eggs in a large saucepan and add cold water to cover. Bring to a boil over high heat. Cover, remove from the heat, and let stand for 15 minutes. Drain off the water, then fill the saucepan with cold water and let stand for 10 minutes, or until the eggs have cooled. Shell the eggs and discard 2 of the yolks. Chop the eggs and place in a medium bowl. Stir in the beans, celery, cucumber, apricots, onion, yogurt, mayonnaise, cilantro, lemon juice, and curry powder.

2. Divide the spinach among 4 plates and top each with one-quarter of the egg salad. Serve.

Per serving: 222 calories, 5 g fat, 1 g saturated fat, 17 g protein, 29 g carbohydrates, 9 g fiber, 325 mg sodium

MAKE IT A SALT SOLUTION MEAL
Boil ½ cup frozen edamame in pods, and serve warm (322 calories and 330 mg sodium total).

Three-Bean Salad

Prep time: 5 minutes ⁝▹ **Cook time:** 2 minutes ⁝▹ **Total time:** 1 hour 7 minutes
⁝▹ MAKES 4 SERVINGS

8 ounces green beans, trimmed and halved crosswise

4 ounces yellow wax beans, trimmed and halved crosswise

1½ cups no-salt-added red kidney beans, rinsed and drained

4 ounces firm tofu, drained, cut into ½" cubes

1 large tomato, chopped

½ hothouse cucumber, chopped

½ small red onion, chopped

1 tablespoon extra virgin olive oil

2 tablespoons balsamic vinegar

1 tablespoon chopped fresh basil or ½ teaspoon dried

1 tablespoon chopped fresh parsley

¼ teaspoon salt

⅛ teaspoon ground black pepper

1. Bring a large pot of water to a boil over high heat. Add the green beans and wax beans. Return to a boil and cook for 2 minutes, or until the beans are crisp-tender.

2. Drain and rinse under cold water to stop the cooking. Drain again, then transfer to a large bowl.

3. Stir in the kidney beans, tofu, tomato, cucumber, onion, oil, vinegar, basil, parsley, salt, and pepper. Cover and refrigerate for 1 hour before serving.

Per serving: 210 calories, 7 g fat, 1 g saturated fat, 13 g protein, 26 g carbohydrates, 12 g fiber, 171 mg sodium

MAKE IT A SALT SOLUTION MEAL
Serve with 1 slice whole grain bread (280 calories and 303 mg sodium total).

Couscous and Lentil Salad

Prep time: 10 minutes ⁞▷ **Cook time:** 20 minutes ⁞▷ **Total time:** 30 minutes ⁞▷ MAKES 4 SERVINGS

³/₄ cup brown lentils, rinsed

2 tablespoons balsamic vinegar

³/₄ cup water

¹/₂ cup couscous

¹/₈ + ¹/₄ teaspoon salt

3 cups fresh spinach

1 medium red bell pepper, chopped

¹/₂ cup chopped red onion

2 ribs celery, chopped

3 tablespoons chopped fresh basil

2 tablespoons extra virgin olive oil

1. Place the lentils in a small saucepan and add enough water to cover by 2". Bring to a simmer over medium heat and simmer until the lentils are tender but still hold their shape, 18 to 20 minutes. Drain, transfer to a bowl, and stir in 2 teaspoons of the vinegar. Cool. Meanwhile, bring the water to a boil in a small saucepan over medium-high heat. Stir in the couscous and ¹/₈ teaspoon of salt. Cover, remove from the heat, and let stand for 5 minutes. Fluff with a fork and cool for 10 minutes. Transfer to the bowl with the lentils.

2. To the cool lentil mixture, add the spinach, bell pepper, onion, celery, and basil and stir. Add the remaining 4 teaspoons vinegar, the oil, and ¹/₄ teaspoon of salt. Mix well.

Per serving: 295 calories, 8 g fat, 1 g saturated fat, 14 g protein, 44 g carbohydrates, 11 g fiber, 260 mg sodium

Nutty Fruit Salad

Prep time: 15 minutes ⁙ **Total time:** 15 minutes ⁙ MAKES 4 SERVINGS

 3 cups shredded iceberg lettuce
 3 cups mixed spring greens
 2 medium pears, sliced (about
  1½ cups)
1½ cups diced fresh pineapple
 1 blood or navel orange, peeled and
  sectioned

¼ cup dried cranberries or raisins
¼ cup sliced natural almonds
 5 tablespoons coarsely chopped
  Brazil nuts
⅓ cup light raspberry vinaigrette

In a large bowl, combine the iceberg lettuce, greens, pears, pineapple, and orange.
Sprinkle with the cranberries or raisins, almonds, and Brazil nuts, and drizzle with
the vinaigrette. Toss well.

Per serving: 236 calories, 9 g fat, 2 g saturated fat, 4 g protein, 38 g carbohydrates, 7 g fiber,
41 mg sodium

MAKE IT A SALT SOLUTION MEAL
Serve with ½ cup soymilk (286 calories and 101 mg sodium total).

Middle Eastern Chopped Salad

Prep time: 25 minutes ⁘ **Total time:** 25 minutes ⁘ MAKES 4 SERVINGS

5 teaspoons extra virgin olive oil

2 tablespoons red wine vinegar

1 clove garlic, minced

$\frac{1}{8}$ teaspoon salt

$\frac{1}{4}$ teaspoon ground black pepper

3 tomatoes

1 cucumber, peeled and seeded

1 red bell pepper

1 green bell pepper

12 ounces cooked boneless, skinless chicken breast

$\frac{1}{4}$ red onion, finely chopped

2 tablespoons chopped parsley

2 tablespoons crumbled feta cheese

2 whole wheat pitas (6")

1. In a large bowl, whisk together the oil, vinegar, garlic, salt, and black pepper. Set aside.

2. Seed the tomatoes and coarsely chop. Chop the cucumber, bell peppers, and chicken into similar-size pieces.

3. Add the vegetables and chicken to the oil mixture along with the onion, parsley, and feta. Divide among 4 bowls.

4. Toast the pitas and cut each into 4 wedges. Serve 2 wedges per person.

Per serving: 311 calories, 11 g fat, 3 g saturated fat, 31 g protein, 22 g carbohydrates, 5 g fiber, 317 mg sodium

Healthy Hamburger and Veggie Soup

Prep time: 15 minutes ⁑ **Cook time:** 30 minutes ⁑ **Total time:** 45 minutes ⁑ MAKES 4 SERVINGS

3/4 pound ground beef sirloin
1 medium onion, chopped
1 teaspoon dried Italian seasoning
1/2 teaspoon ground black pepper
1 can (14 1/2 ounces) unsalted diced tomatoes
3 cups low-sodium fat-free beef broth

3/4 cup reduced-sodium tomato juice
1 cup frozen mixed peas and carrots
1 cup frozen cut green beans
1 cup frozen baby lima beans
1 cup frozen corn kernels
1/2 cup cooked brown rice
4 cups chopped fresh spinach
1 tablespoon Worcestershire sauce

1. In a medium nonstick skillet over medium-high heat, crumble the ground sirloin. Sprinkle in the onion, Italian seasoning, and pepper. Cook, breaking up the beef with the back of a spoon, for about 10 minutes, or until the beef is browned. Drain in a colander, if necessary.

2. Transfer to a Dutch oven. Stir the tomatoes (with their juice), broth, tomato juice, peas and carrots, green beans, lima beans, corn, and rice into the beef. Bring to a boil over high heat. Reduce the heat to low, cover, and simmer about 20 minutes, or until the vegetables are tender and the flavors have blended. Stir in the spinach and Worcestershire sauce and cook for 1 to 2 minutes, stirring, until the spinach has wilted.

Per serving: 326 calories, 6 g fat, 2 g saturated fat, 29 g protein, 41 g carbohydrates, 8 g fiber, 290 mg sodium

Minestrone Soup

Prep time: 15 minutes ⫸ **Cook time:** 50 minutes ⫸ **Total time:** 1 hour 5 minutes ⫸ MAKES 4 SERVINGS

1 tablespoon extra virgin olive oil
1 medium onion, chopped
3 cloves garlic, minced
3 large ribs celery, cut into 1/4" dice
2 carrots, cut into 1/4" dice
1 teaspoon dried oregano
8 ounces zucchini (1 medium), cut into 1/4" dice
8 ounces yellow squash (1 medium), cut into 1/4" dice

4 cups low-sodium chicken broth
1/8 teaspoon salt
2 cans (14 1/2 ounces) no-salt-added diced tomatoes
4 ounces tubetti pasta
1 can (15 ounces) no-salt-added cannellini beans, drained and rinsed

Heat the oil in a Dutch oven over medium-high heat. Add the onion, garlic, celery, carrots, and oregano. Cook, stirring occasionally, until beginning to soften, 3 to 5 minutes. Add the zucchini and squash. Cook until starting to soften, 4 to 5 minutes. Pour in the broth, salt, and tomatoes, and bring to a boil. Reduce the heat to medium-low and simmer, covered, until the vegetables are crisp-tender, about 20 minutes. Stir in the pasta, cover, and simmer until cooked, 10 to 12 minutes. Stir in the beans and cook until heated through, 2 to 3 minutes longer.

Per serving: 304 calories, 5 g fat, 1 g saturated fat, 14 g protein, 51 g carbohydrates, 9 g fiber, 297 mg sodium

Tofu Split Pea Soup

Prep time: 15 minutes · **Cook time:** 1 hour 13 minutes · **Total time:** 1 hour 28 minutes
· MAKES 4 SERVINGS

4 slices lower-sodium bacon,
chopped
2 medium onions, chopped
1 cup chopped carrot
1 cup chopped celery
4 cloves garlic, minced
1 teaspoon chopped fresh thyme

1 cup yellow split peas
3 cups low-sodium chicken broth
2 cups water
4 ounces tofu, well drained
$\frac{1}{8}$ teaspoon salt
$\frac{1}{4}$ teaspoon ground black pepper

1. Heat a Dutch oven over medium-high heat. Add the bacon and cook, stirring occasionally, until browned, about 4 to 5 minutes. Stir in the onions, carrot, celery, garlic, and thyme. Cook, stirring occasionally, until starting to soften, about 5 to 6 minutes. Add the split peas, broth, and water. Bring to a boil, reduce the heat to medium-low, partially cover, and simmer until the split peas are very tender, about 1 hour. Remove from the heat and cool for 10 minutes.

2. In batches, transfer the soup to a blender, add the tofu, and puree. Return the soup to the Dutch oven and cook over medium heat for 1 to 2 minutes, or until heated through. Remove from the heat and stir in the salt and pepper.

Per serving: 327 calories, 7 g fat, 2 g saturated fat, 24 g protein, 45 g carbohydrates, 16 g fiber, 274 mg sodium

Tuscan Bean Stew

Prep time: 10 minutes ⁞▸ **Cook time:** 15 minutes ⁞▸ **Total time:** 25 minutes ⁞▸ MAKES 8 SERVINGS

2 teaspoons olive oil

1½ cups finely chopped fresh fennel or anise

¼ pound Italian sausage, crumbled

1 tablespoon finely minced garlic

3 cups fat-free reduced-sodium chicken broth

3 cups dried small white or navy beans, rinsed and soaked overnight and drained

1 teaspoon dried basil

2 ripe plum tomatoes, chopped

½ cup thinly sliced fresh basil leaves

1. Heat the oil in a 6-quart pressure cooker over medium heat.

2. Add the fennel or anise and sausage and cover with the lid, but do not lock. Cook for 4 minutes, or until the fennel or anise is tender and the sausage is browned. Add the garlic and cook for 1 minute. Add the broth, beans, and basil. Cover with the lid, lock in position, and bring to full pressure over high heat (high pressure on those models with a choice). Reduce the heat slightly to moderate steam (detailed directions will be with your cooker). Cook for 10 minutes.

3. Switch the pressure indicator to quick release or run cold water over the lid to reduce the pressure. (See the manufacturer's directions for the quick release of steam or temperature cooldown.) Unlock the lid. Puree ⅔ cup of the stew in a blender and return to the pot. Stir in the tomatoes and fresh basil.

Per serving: 315 calories, 3 g fat, 0 g saturated fat, 21 g protein, 53 g carbohydrates, 21 g fiber, 297 mg sodium

DINNERS

Spice-Rubbed Chicken with Watermelon Salad

Prep time: 15 minutes ⋙ **Cook time:** 26 minutes ⋙ **Total time:** 41 minutes ⋙ MAKES 4 SERVINGS

- 2 teaspoons packed light brown sugar
- 1 teaspoon paprika
- $\frac{1}{2}$ teaspoon garlic powder
- $\frac{1}{2}$ teaspoon ground cumin
- $\frac{1}{4}$ teaspoon dried thyme
- $\frac{1}{4}$ teaspoon salt
- $\frac{1}{8}$ teaspoon ground black pepper

- 4 (6 ounce) bone-in, skinless chicken thighs, ($1\frac{1}{2}$ pounds), trimmed of all visible fat
- 5 cups watermelon cubes
- 4 cups fresh arugula leaves, torn
- 4 cups fresh baby spinach
- $\frac{1}{2}$ cup thinly sliced red onion
- 3 tablespoons fresh lemon juice
- 2 teaspoons honey

1. Coat the grill rack with cooking spray. Prepare the grill for medium-hot indirect-heat grilling.

2. In a small bowl, combine the sugar, paprika, garlic powder, cumin, thyme, $\frac{1}{8}$ teaspoon of the salt, and the pepper. Rub the mixture over the chicken thighs. Place the chicken on the grill rack, away from the heat source. Cover the grill and cook the chicken, turning once, until a thermometer inserted into the thickest part of the thigh registers 165°F, about 24 to 26 minutes.

3. Meanwhile, in a large bowl, combine the watermelon, arugula, spinach, onion, lemon juice, honey, and the remaining $\frac{1}{8}$ teaspoon salt. Serve with the chicken.

Per serving: 290 calories, 11 g fat, 3 g saturated fat, 27 g protein, 24 g carbohydrates, 2 g fiber, 258 mg sodium

Cilantro-Chicken Stir-Fry

Prep time: 15 minutes ▷ **Cook time:** 32 minutes ▷ **Total time:** 47 minutes ▷ MAKES 4 SERVINGS

½ cup quinoa, rinsed under cold
  water and drained
1 cup water
1 medium sweet potato (8 ounces),
  peeled and cut into ¼" cubes
4 teaspoons canola oil
12 ounces boneless, skinless chicken
  breast, cut into ½" cubes
1 medium onion, chopped

1 jalapeño chile pepper, seeded and
  finely chopped (wear plastic gloves
  when handling)
1 medium red bell pepper, chopped
1 clove garlic, minced
1 teaspoon ground cumin
1 cup frozen or fresh peas
3 tablespoons chopped fresh cilantro
¼ teaspoon salt
⅛ teaspoon ground black pepper

1. In a small saucepan over medium-high heat, combine the quinoa and water. Bring to a boil, reduce the heat to medium, and simmer until the liquid has been absorbed, about 12 to 15 minutes. Meanwhile, place the sweet potato in a small saucepan and add enough cold water to cover by 2". Bring to a boil over medium-high heat and cook until just tender, about 3 to 4 minutes. Drain and set aside.

2. Heat 2 teaspoons of the oil in a large nonstick skillet over medium-high heat. Add the chicken and cook, stirring occasionally, until starting to brown, about 4 minutes. Transfer to a bowl and set aside. Return the skillet to the heat and add the remaining 2 teaspoons oil. Stir in the onion and jalapeño pepper. Cook, stirring occasionally, for 1 minute. Add the bell pepper, garlic, and cumin, and cook until starting to soften, 2 to 3 minutes. Stir in the peas and reserved chicken and cook for 2 minutes. Add the quinoa and reserved sweet potato. Cook, stirring often, until hot, about 1 to 2 minutes. Off the heat, stir in the cilantro, salt, and pepper.

Per serving: 307 calories, 8 g fat, 1 g saturated fat, 24 g protein, 34 g carbohydrates, 6 g fiber, 264 mg sodium

Indian-Style Chicken

Prep time: 19 minutes ⊳• **Cook time:** 16 minutes ⊳• **Total time:** 1 hour 5 minutes
⊳• MAKES 4 SERVINGS

4 (6-ounce) bone-in chicken thighs, skin removed

¾ cups plain yogurt

1 tablespoon fresh lemon juice

1 tablespoon grated fresh ginger

2 cloves garlic, minced

1½ teaspoons ground coriander

1½ teaspoons paprika

¾ teaspoon ground cumin

¼ teaspoon salt

¼ teaspoon crushed red-pepper flakes

1. With a sharp knife, cut three or four ¼"-deep slashes in each piece of chicken. In a large bowl, combine the yogurt, lemon juice, ginger, garlic, coriander, paprika, cumin, salt, and red-pepper flakes. Stir until well combined. Add the chicken to the bowl and turn to coat well with the marinade.

2. Marinate the chicken for 30 minutes at room temperature or refrigerate, covered, up to 24 hours. (If the chicken is refrigerated, remove it about 30 minutes before cooking.)

3. Coat the broiler pan with cooking spray. Heat the broiler. With tongs, pick up one piece of chicken at a time and let any excess marinade drip back into the bowl. Set the chicken on the broiler pan. Discard the marinade.

4. Broil the chicken about 6" from the heat source until brown, about 8 minutes. Turn the thighs over and broil 6 to 8 minutes longer, or until a thermometer inserted into the thickest portion registers 175°F. Remove from the oven.

Per serving: 240 calories, 7 g fat, 2 g saturated fat, 37 g protein, 6 g carbohydrates, 1 g fiber, 329 mg sodium

MAKE IT A SALT SOLUTION MEAL
Serve with ¼ cup whole wheat couscous (303 calories and 331 mg sodium total).

Chicken Picadillo

Prep time: 8 minutes ⁑ **Cook time:** 11 minutes ⁑ **Total time:** 19 minutes ⁑ MAKES 4 SERVINGS

½ pound boneless, skinless chicken thighs, trimmed of all visible fat

2 teaspoons olive oil

½ large red bell pepper, finely chopped

1 onion, finely chopped

2 cloves garlic, minced

¼ teaspoon salt

1 cup canned no-salt-added diced tomatoes

6 tablespoons raisins

¼ cup chopped blanched Brazil nuts

2 tablespoons chopped fresh cilantro

2 cups hot cooked long-grain brown rice

1. Cut the chicken into chunks. Place in a food processor and pulse 8 times to chop coarsely. (The chicken can also be chopped by hand with a large heavy knife.)

2. Heat the oil in a large nonstick skillet over medium-high heat. Add the bell pepper, onion, garlic, and salt. Cook, stirring, for 2 minutes, or until the vegetables are sizzling and the garlic is fragrant.

3. Add the chicken. Cook, stirring, for 3 minutes, or until the chicken is just beginning to brown.

4. Add the tomatoes and raisins. Reduce the heat and simmer for 5 minutes, or until the chicken is cooked through. Stir in the nuts and cilantro. Serve over the rice.

Per serving: 326 calories, 11 g fat, 2 g saturated fat, 17 g protein, 42 g carbohydrates, 5 g fiber, 228 mg sodium

Salsa Chicken Stir-Fry

Prep time: 10 minutes   **Cook time:** 12 minutes   **Total time:** 22 minutes   MAKES 4 SERVINGS

1 tablespoon olive oil

1 pound boneless, skinless chicken breasts, cut into thin strips

½ onion, thinly sliced

1 clove garlic, minced

½ medium red bell pepper, thinly sliced

1 cup broccoli florets

¾ cup prepared salsa

⅛ teaspoon ground black pepper

¼ teaspoon crushed red-pepper flakes (optional)

2 cups hot cooked brown rice

1. Heat the oil in a large nonstick skillet over medium heat. Add the chicken and cook, stirring frequently, until it is no longer pink and the juices run clear, about 8 to 10 minutes. Remove the chicken from the pan.

2. In the same pan, cook the onion, garlic, bell pepper, and broccoli for 6 to 7 minutes, or until crisp-tender.

3. Return the chicken to the pan. Add the salsa and stir to coat. Cook for 1 to 2 minutes, or until heated through. Stir in the black pepper and red-pepper flakes, if using. Serve over the brown rice.

Per serving: 303 calories, 6 g fat, 1 g saturated fat, 31 g protein, 30 g carbohydrates, 4 g fiber, 296 mg sodium

Chicken Cacciatore

Prep time: 10 minutes ⁘ **Cook time:** 15 minutes ⁘ **Total time:** 25 minutes ⁘ MAKES 4 SERVINGS

1 pound boneless, skinless chicken
breast tenders

2 teaspoons olive oil

1 package (8 ounces) cremini
mushrooms, quartered

$\frac{1}{2}$ medium red bell pepper,
cut into strips

1 small onion, chopped

2 cloves garlic, minced

$\frac{1}{4}$ teaspoon ground black pepper

1 can (14$\frac{1}{2}$ ounces) no-salt-added
diced tomatoes with basil, garlic,
and oregano

4 ounces multigrain rotini pasta

20 pitted large black olives

1 tablespoon minced parsley

1. Bring a medium pot of water to a boil over high heat. Meanwhile, cut the chicken into $\frac{1}{2}$" pieces.

2. Heat the oil in a large nonstick skillet over medium-high heat. Add the chicken and cook, turning occasionally, for 4 minutes, or until browned on all sides. Transfer to a plate.

3. Add the mushrooms, bell pepper, onion, garlic, and black pepper to the skillet and toss to combine.

4. Reduce the heat to medium, cover, and cook, tossing occasionally, for 3 minutes, or until the mushrooms exude liquid. Uncover and cook to evaporate most of the liquid, about 8 minutes.

5. Add the tomatoes and the reserved chicken with any accumulated juices from the plate. Reduce the heat to a simmer.

6. When the water boils, add the pasta and cook according to package directions. Drain the pasta and transfer to the skillet. Add the olives and toss gently to combine. Serve sprinkled with the parsley.

Per serving: 330 calories, 8 g fat, 1 g saturated fat, 32 g protein, 34 g carbohydrates, 6 g fiber, 296 mg sodium

Tomato-Topped
Turkey Meat Loaf

Prep time: 15 minutes ⋅ **Cook time:** 58 minutes ⋅ **Total time:** 1 hour 23 minutes
⋅ MAKES 6 SERVINGS

2 teaspoons olive oil

½ cup chopped onion

2 cloves garlic, minced

3 cups spinach, chopped

2 cups kale, chopped

12 ounces lean ground turkey

12 ounces ground turkey breast

½ cup plain dried bread crumbs

1 large egg

¾ cup low-sodium ketchup

¼ teaspoon salt

1. Preheat the oven to 350°F. Coat a large baking sheet with cooking spray.

2. Heat the oil in a large nonstick skillet over medium-high heat. Add the onion and garlic. Cook, stirring occasionally, until starting to soften, about 2 minutes. Stir in the spinach and kale. Cook, stirring often, until very tender, about 4 to 5 minutes. Transfer to a bowl and cool completely.

3. Combine the turkey, turkey breast, bread crumbs, egg, ¼ cup of the ketchup, the cooled spinach mixture, and salt in a large bowl and mix well. Transfer the mixture to the prepared baking sheet and form into a loaf 8" long x 1¾" high x 4" wide. Spread the top with the remaining ½ cup ketchup.

4. Bake until a thermometer inserted into the center of the meat loaf registers 165°F, about 48 to 50 minutes. Cool for 10 minutes before slicing.

Per serving: 259 calories, 8 g fat, 2 g saturated fat, 28 g protein, 18 g carbohydrates, 2 g fiber, 284 mg sodium

MAKE IT A SALT SOLUTION MEAL
Serve with 1 small baked sweet potato sprinkled with cinnamon or nutmeg (313 calories and 306 mg sodium total).

Rosemary Salmon

Prep time: 5 minutes ❧ **Cook time:** 30 minutes ❧ **Total time:** 35 minutes ❧ MAKES 4 SERVINGS

4 (4-ounce) salmon fillets
4 sprigs rosemary
¼ cup lemon juice
¼ teaspoon salt

¼ teaspoon ground black pepper
1 package (10 ounces) frozen
  chopped spinach, thawed
½ cup hot cooked brown rice

1. Preheat the grill to high.

2. Place each salmon fillet on a piece of foil. Sprinkle each with 1 sprig rosemary and 1 tablespoon lemon juice and season with the salt and pepper. Fold the foil over the fish and wrap tightly, crimping the sides as you go to form a packet. Place the fish on the grill and cook for 9 to 12 minutes.

3. Remove from the grill when the packets have puffed up. Open the packets very carefully as they will release a lot of steam. The fish is done when it is opaque.

4. Meanwhile, heat the spinach according to package directions. Serve the salmon over the spinach and with the rice.

Per serving: 319 calories, 13 g fat, 3 g saturated fat, 27 g protein, 22 g carbohydrates, 4 g fiber, 269 mg sodium

Halibut Steaks with Onions and Peppers

Prep time: 5 minutes ❧ **Cook time:** 20 minutes ❧ **Total time:** 1 hour 25 minutes
❧ MAKES 4 SERVINGS

2 tablespoons lemon juice
¼ teaspoon salt
½ teaspoon paprika
4 (6-ounce) halibut steaks
1 tablespoon olive oil

½ cup chopped onion
1 large red bell pepper, cut into strips
1 large green bell pepper, cut into strips

1. In a shallow bowl, combine the lemon juice, salt, and paprika. Add the fish, cover, and refrigerate for 1 hour, turning once.

2. Preheat the oven to 450°F. Coat an 11" × 7" baking dish with cooking spray.

3. Heat the oil in a medium skillet over medium-high heat. Add the onion and bell peppers and cook, stirring occasionally, for about 5 to 7 minutes, or until the onions are brown.

4. Place the fish in the prepared baking dish and top with the onion and bell pepper strips. Bake for 10 minutes, or until the fish is just opaque.

Per serving: 240 calories, 7 g fat, 1 g saturated fat, 36 g protein, 5 g carbohydrates, 1 g fiber, 240 mg sodium

MAKE IT A SALT SOLUTION MEAL
Serve with 2 cups spinach, sautéed until soft in 1 teaspoon olive oil (294 calories and 287 mg sodium total).

Home-Style Beef Stew

Prep time: 23 minutes · **Cook time:** 2 hours 20 minutes · **Total time:** 2 hours 43 minutes · MAKES 4 SERVINGS

2 teaspoons olive oil

2 tablespoons all-purpose flour

1/4 teaspoon salt

1/4 teaspoon ground black pepper

10 ounces lean boneless beef round steak, trimmed of all visible fat and cut into 1" cubes

3/4 cup frozen pearl onions

3 cloves garlic, minced

1/4 teaspoon dried thyme

1/4 cup dry red wine

1 cup water

3 tablespoons tomato paste

1 3/4 cups low-sodium beef broth

6 ounces baby red potatoes, quartered (about 6 potatoes or 1 1/2 cups)

12 baby carrots

12 baby pattypan squash, halved

8 ounces fresh mushrooms, sliced

1/4 cup chopped fresh parsley

1. Warm 1 teaspoon of the oil in a Dutch oven over medium-high heat. In a medium bowl, combine the flour, salt, and pepper.

2. Working in batches, dredge the beef in the flour mixture, add to the Dutch oven, and cook for 3 to 4 minutes, or until browned on all sides. Do not overcrowd the pan. Using a slotted spoon, transfer the beef to a plate.

3. Add the remaining 1 teaspoon oil to the Dutch oven. Reduce the heat to medium and add the onions, garlic, and thyme. Cook, stirring often, for 6 to 7 minutes, or until the onions are slightly softened.

4. Stir in the wine, water, and tomato paste. Using a wooden spoon, scrape up any browned bits from the bottom of the pan.

5. Add the broth and beef. Increase the heat to medium-high and bring to a boil. Reduce the heat to medium, partially cover, and simmer for 1 hour, or until the beef is tender.

6. Add the potatoes and carrots. Simmer for 20 minutes.

7. Add the squash, mushrooms, and parsley. Simmer for 10 minutes, or until the vegetables are tender.

Per serving: 326 calories, 11 g fat, 4 g saturated fat, 26 g protein, 27 g carbohydrates, 4 g fiber, 249 mg sodium

THE SALT SOLUTION RECIPES

Penne Bolognese

Prep time: 10 minutes ⏵ **Cook time:** 35 minutes ⏵ **Total time:** 45 minutes ⏵ MAKES 4 SERVINGS

6 ounces whole wheat penne
8 ounces extra-lean ground beef
1 medium onion, chopped
2 cloves garlic, minced
¼ cup finely chopped carrot
1 teaspoon dried oregano
1 medium zucchini (8 ounces), trimmed and chopped

1 can (14½ ounces) unsalted diced tomatoes
½ cup unsalted tomato paste
¼ cup water
¼ teaspoon salt
3 tablespoons reduced-fat mozzarella cheese

1. Bring a large pot of water to a boil over high heat. Add the penne and cook according to package directions and drain.

2. Meanwhile, heat a large nonstick skillet over medium-high heat. Add the beef and cook, breaking it into smaller pieces, until no longer pink, about 3 to 4 minutes. Stir in the onion, garlic, carrot, and oregano. Cook, stirring occasionally, until starting to soften, about 2 minutes. Add the zucchini and cook until starting to soften, about 2 minutes. Stir in the tomatoes, tomato paste, and water. Bring to a boil, reduce the heat to medium, and simmer until slightly thickened, about 12 to 15 minutes. Remove from the heat and stir in the salt. Serve over the pasta, and sprinkle the cheese on top.

Per serving: 302 calories, 4 g fat, 2 g saturated fat, 22 g protein, 48 g carbohydrates, 9 g fiber, 268 mg sodium

Pork Tenderloin with Avocado Salad

Prep time: 15 minutes ⁛ **Cook time:** 25 minutes ⁛ **Total time:** 50 minutes ⁛ MAKES 4 SERVINGS

2 teaspoons packed light brown sugar

1 teaspoon chili powder

1 teaspoon ground cumin

$\frac{1}{4}$ teaspoon garlic powder

$\frac{1}{4}$ + $\frac{1}{8}$ teaspoon salt

$\frac{1}{4}$ teaspoon ground black pepper

1 pound well-trimmed pork tenderloin

1 cucumber, peeled and halved lengthwise and cut into $\frac{1}{2}$" slices

2 tomatoes, cut into 1" chunks

$\frac{1}{2}$ Hass avocado, cut into 1" chunks

1 small white onion, thinly sliced

1 tablespoon olive oil

1 tablespoon fresh lime juice

4 corn tortillas (6" diameter)

1. Coat the grill rack with cooking spray. Preheat the grill to medium-high.

2. In a small bowl, combine the brown sugar, chili powder, cumin, garlic powder, $\frac{1}{4}$ teaspoon of salt, and the pepper. Rub the mixture over the pork. Set the pork on the grill rack. Grill, turning occasionally, for 22 to 24 minutes, or until a thermometer inserted in the center of the pork registers 155°F.

3. Transfer to a cutting board and let rest for 10 minutes.

4. In a bowl, combine the cucumber, tomatoes, avocado, onion, oil, lime juice, and remaining $\frac{1}{8}$ teaspoon salt.

5. Warm the tortillas on the grill for 30 seconds per side. Slice the pork and serve with the avocado salad and tortillas.

Per serving: 273 calories, 10 g fat, 2 g saturated fat, 27 g protein, 20 g carbohydrates, 4 g fiber, 297 mg sodium

Pork and Sweet Potato Skillet

Prep time: 14 minutes ❧ **Cook time:** 11 minutes ❧ **Total time:** 25 minutes ❧ MAKES 4 SERVINGS

3 teaspoons olive oil

1 pound well-trimmed pork tenderloin, cut into 1" pieces

2 large sweet potatoes, cut into ½" pieces

1 red onion, cut into ½" pieces

1 red bell pepper, cut into ½" pieces

¾ cup water

1 tablespoon honey

1 chipotle chile pepper in adobo sauce, minced

Juice of 1 lime

1 Hass avocado, pitted and peeled

¼ cup chopped fresh cilantro

1 tablespoon chopped yellow or white onion

¼ teaspoon salt

1. Heat 1 teaspoon of the oil in a large nonstick skillet over medium-high heat. Add the pork and cook for 5 to 7 minutes, or until browned. Transfer to a plate and keep warm.

2. Add the sweet potatoes, red onion, bell pepper, and ½ cup of the water to the skillet. Cover and cook for 5 minutes, or until the sweet potatoes are tender.

3. Remove from the heat and stir in the honey, chipotle pepper, and half of the lime juice. Return the pork to the skillet and toss to combine.

4. In a blender, place the avocado, 2 tablespoons of the cilantro, the onion, salt, and the remaining lime juice, the remaining ¼ cup water, and the remaining 2 teaspoons oil. Process for 1 minute to make a sauce.

5. Serve the pork and vegetables sprinkled with the remaining cilantro and the avocado sauce on the side.

Per serving: 302 calories, 11 g fat, 2 g saturated fat, 26 g protein, 24 g carbohydrates, 1 g fiber, 264 mg sodium

Apricot-Ginger Glazed Pork Tenderloin with Succotash

Prep time: 15 minutes ⋗ **Cook time:** 24 minutes ⋗ **Total time:** 39 minutes ⋗ MAKES 4 SERVINGS

PORK

- ¼ cup apricot preserves
- 1 tablespoon grated fresh ginger
- 1 pound lean pork tenderloin, trimmed of all visible fat
- ⅛ teaspoon salt
- ¼ teaspoon ground black pepper

SUCCOTASH

- 1 teaspoon extra virgin olive oil
- ½ medium onion, chopped
- 1 package (10 ounces) frozen cut okra
- 1 teaspoon dried oregano
- 1 cup fresh or frozen corn kernels
- 2 teaspoons cider vinegar
- 1 teaspoon sugar
- 3 tablespoons thinly sliced fresh basil
- ¼ teaspoon salt

1. Coat the grill rack with cooking spray. Preheat the grill for medium-hot cooking.

2. In a small bowl, combine the preserves and ginger. Sprinkle the pork with the salt and pepper and set on the grill rack. Close the cover and grill the pork for 10 minutes, then turn and grill for 10 minutes longer. Brush the pork with half of the preserves mixture. Grill for 2 minutes, turn, and brush with the remaining preserves mixture. Grill for 2 minutes longer, or until a thermometer inserted into the thickest portion of the pork registers 155°F. Turn the pork and grill for 30 seconds to set the glaze. Transfer to a cutting board, cover loosely with foil, and let stand for 10 minutes before slicing. Cut into 16 slices.

3. Meanwhile, heat the oil in a large nonstick skillet over medium-high heat. Add the onion, okra, and oregano and cook, stirring occasionally, until the onion starts to brown and the okra stops giving off liquid, about 6 to 7 minutes. Stir in the corn and cook until it starts to brown slightly, about 3 minutes. Add the vinegar and sugar and cook for 1 minute. Remove from the heat and stir in the basil and salt. Serve with the sliced pork.

Per serving: 251 calories, 5 g fat, 1 g saturated fat, 25 g protein, 29 g carbohydrates, 3 g fiber, 279 mg sodium

MAKE IT A SALT SOLUTION MEAL
Serve with ⅓ cup cooked whole wheat couscous (309 calories and 303 mg sodium total).

Vegetable Penne

Prep time: 10 minutes ⁂ **Cook time:** 24 minutes ⁂ **Total time:** 34 minutes ⁂ MAKES 4 SERVINGS

3 cups broccoli florets	1 cup sliced fennel
6 ounces penne	2 cups grape tomatoes, halved
1 tablespoon extra virgin olive oil	1 can (15 ounces) no-salt-added
1 medium onion, sliced	chickpeas, rinsed and drained
2 cloves garlic, minced	$\frac{1}{4}$ teaspoon salt
1 teaspoon dried basil	$\frac{1}{4}$ teaspoon ground black pepper

1. Bring a large pot of water to a boil over high heat. Add the broccoli, return to a boil, and cook for 2 minutes. Remove with a slotted spoon and transfer to a bowl. Return the water to a boil, add the penne, and cook according to package directions and drain.

2. Heat the oil in a large nonstick skillet over medium-high heat. Add the onion, garlic, and basil. Cook until starting to soften about 2 minutes. Stir in the fennel and cook for 2 minutes. Add the tomatoes and cook until starting to wilt, 2 to 3 minutes. Add the chickpeas and cook for 2 minutes. Stir in the broccoli and cook until hot, 2 minutes. Remove from the heat and stir in the salt and pepper. Toss with the penne and serve.

Per serving: 317 calories, 5 g fat, 1 g saturated fat, 13 g protein, 57 g carbohydrates, 8 g fiber, 197 mg sodium

Angel Hair Pasta with Fresh Tomato Sauce

Prep time: 4 hours 25 minutes ▷ **Cook time:** 10 minutes ▷ **Total time:** 4 hours 35 minutes
▷ MAKES 4 SERVINGS

6 medium tomatoes, chopped	1 clove garlic, minced
½ onion, chopped	½ teaspoon sugar
½ bunch fresh basil, thinly sliced, + extra basil for garnish	6 ounces angel hair pasta
¼ cup red wine vinegar	4 ounces shredded reduced-fat mozzarella cheese
1 tablespoon olive oil	

1. In a large bowl, combine the tomatoes, onion, basil, vinegar, oil, garlic, and sugar. Cover the bowl with plastic wrap and let it stand at room temperature for at least 4 hours.

2. When the sauce is ready, cook the pasta according to package directions and drain. Transfer the pasta to a large serving bowl, and cover with the sauce and cheese. Gently toss to mix well.

Per serving: 296 calories, 9 g fat, 3 g saturated fat, 16 g protein, 42 g carbohydrates, 5 g fiber, 215 mg sodium

Lentil Quinoa Burgers

Prep time: 17 minutes ⊪ **Cook time:** 33 minutes ⊪ **Total time:** 50 minutes ⊪ MAKES 6 SERVINGS

½ cup quinoa

1 cup water

1 can (19 ounces) lentils, rinsed and drained

½ cup plain soft white bread crumbs, toasted

1 egg, lightly beaten

2 cloves garlic, chopped

2 teaspoons ground cumin

⅓ cup cilantro

Juice of ½ lemon

Salt

Ground black pepper

⅓ cup walnut pieces

2 teaspoons butter

8 ounces cremini mushrooms, sliced

¼ cup dry red wine

2 teaspoons vegetable oil

6 reduced-calorie hamburger rolls

1. In a saucepan, combine the quinoa and water. Bring to a boil and simmer for about 10 minutes, or until the water has evaporated. Let the quinoa cool.

2. In a bowl, combine half the lentils, the bread crumbs, egg, garlic, cumin, cilantro, lemon juice, cooked quinoa, and salt and pepper to taste. Place in a food processor or blender and process until well combined. Add the remaining lentils and the walnuts and pulse until they're incorporated.

3. Form into 6 patties. Preheat the grill to medium. Meanwhile, melt the butter in a skillet over medium heat. Add the mushrooms and cook, stirring regularly, for 5 minutes. Stir in the wine and cook for another 5 minutes. Brush the burgers with the oil and grill for 4 minutes per side.

4. Toast the buns on the grill for 2 minutes. Serve the burgers on the buns and top with the mushrooms.

Per serving: 327 calories, 10 g fat, 2 g saturated fat, 15 g protein, 46 g carbohydrates, 10 g fiber, 240 mg sodium

Black Bean Tacos with Tofu

Prep time: 15 minutes ⫶ **Cook time:** 10 minutes ⫶ **Total time:** 25 minutes ⫶ MAKES 4 SERVINGS

1 cup chopped fresh mango

1 tablespoon chopped fresh cilantro

1 tablespoon fresh lime juice

1 tablespoon olive oil

1 package (14 ounces) firm tofu, drained, pressed, and cut into ½" cubes

1 medium onion, sliced

1 clove garlic, minced

1 teaspoon chili powder

½ teaspoon ground cumin

1 cup no-salt-added black beans, rinsed and drained

¼ teaspoon salt

8 corn tortillas (6" diameter)

1. In a small bowl, combine the mango, cilantro, and lime juice. Set aside.

2. Heat 2 teaspoons of the oil in a large nonstick skillet over medium-high heat. Add the tofu and cook, stirring occasionally, until lightly golden, about 5 to 6 minutes. Transfer the tofu to a plate. Return the skillet to the heat and heat the remaining 1 teaspoon oil. Add the onion, garlic, chili powder, and cumin. Cook until the onion starts to soften, about 2 minutes. Stir in the beans and cook for 1 minute longer. Add the tofu and salt. Cook until hot, about 1 minute.

3. Warm the tortillas according to package directions. Divide the tofu mixture among the tortillas and top each with 2 tablespoons of the mango mixture.

Per serving: 295 calories, 9 g fat, 2 g saturated fat, 15 g protein, 42 g carbohydrates, 8 g fiber, 189 mg sodium

Sweet Potato Vegetarian Shepherd's Pie

Prep time: 15 minutes ⁞▷ **Cook time:** 40 minutes ⁞▷ **Total time:** 55 minutes ⁞▷ MAKES 4 SERVINGS

1 pound orange flesh sweet potatoes, cut into chunks
1½ cups fat-free milk
¼ teaspoon salt
¼ teaspoon ground black pepper
1 tablespoon extra virgin olive oil
1 medium onion, chopped
3 cloves garlic, minced

1 teaspoon chopped fresh thyme
1 package (10 ounces) frozen mixed
vegetables
1½ cups no-salt-added white kidney
beans, rinsed and drained
1½ teaspoons cornstarch
1 teaspoon Worcestershire sauce

1. Place the sweet potatoes in a medium saucepan and add enough cold water to cover by 2". Bring to a boil over medium-high heat and cook until tender, about 10 minutes. Drain and return to the saucepan. Add ½ cup of the milk, ⅛ teaspoon of the salt, and ⅛ teaspoon of the pepper. Mash until smooth and set aside.

2. Preheat the oven to 350°F. Coat a 6-cup baking dish with cooking spray.

3. Meanwhile, heat the oil in a large nonstick skillet over medium-high heat. Stir in the onion, garlic, and thyme. Cook, stirring occasionally, until just starting to brown slightly, about 4 to 5 minutes. Add the mixed vegetables and the beans and cook for 1 minute. In a small bowl, combine the remaining 1 cup milk, ⅛ teaspoon salt, ⅛ teaspoon pepper, the cornstarch, and Worcestershire sauce. Pour into the skillet and cook for 1 minute, or until slightly thickened. Pour the mixture into the prepared baking dish. Spread the top with the mashed sweet potatoes to cover.

4. Bake until the filling is bubbly and the top is very slightly browned, 20 to 22 minutes. Cool for 10 minutes before serving.

Per serving: 320 calories, 4 g fat, 1 g saturated fat, 14 g protein, 60 g carbohydrates, 11 g fiber, 296 mg sodium

Italian Lentil and Broccoli Stew

Prep time: 10 minutes ⁘ **Cook time:** 30 minutes ⁘ **Total time:** 40 minutes ⁘ MAKES 4 SERVINGS

1 small carrot, finely chopped
1 small onion, finely chopped
2 cloves garlic, minced
2 teaspoons olive oil
1 cup dried green or brown lentils
2 cups reduced-sodium vegetable broth or water

1 teaspoon dried oregano
¼ teaspoon ground black pepper
6 cups broccoli florets
16 pitted large green olives, slivered
4 teaspoons shaved or coarsely shredded Parmesan cheese

1. In a medium saucepan, heat the oil over medium heat. Add the carrot, onion, and garlic and cook, stirring occasionally, 4 to 5 minutes, or until the vegetables start to soften.

2. Stir in the lentils, broth or water, oregano, and pepper. Cover and bring to a brisk simmer. Reduce to a low simmer and cook for 20 minutes.

3. Stir in the broccoli. Re-cover and simmer for 5 minutes, or until the lentils are tender and the broccoli is crisp-tender. Stir in the olives. Add more water, if necessary, to thin the stew to the desired consistency.

4. Serve garnished with the cheese.

Per serving: 271 calories, 7 g fat, 1 g saturated fat, 17 g protein, 38 g carbohydrates, 15 g fiber, 313 mg sodium

MAKE IT A SALT SOLUTION MEAL
Serve with a tangerine (280 calories and 310 mg sodium total).

SIDES

Zucchini Chips

Prep time: 8 minutes ❉ **Cook time:** 40 minutes ❉ **Total time:** 48 minutes ❉ MAKES 4 SERVINGS

2 large zucchini, thinkly sliced on the
   diagonal, $\frac{1}{8}$" thick
1 tablespoon olive oil
$\frac{1}{4}$ teaspoon salt
$\frac{1}{4}$ teaspoon garlic powder (optional)

1. Preheat the oven to 400°F.

2. Coat 2 baking sheets with cooking spray. Place the zucchini slices in a large bowl, add the oil, salt, and garlic powder (if using), and toss well. Arrange in a single layer on the baking sheets.

3. Bake, turning often, for 25 minutes. Reduce the oven temperature to 300°F and bake until splotchy brown and crisp, 10 to 15 minutes. Remove to paper towels and let cool. These will keep at room temperature, uncovered, for several hours.

Per serving: 56 calories, 4 g fat, 1 g saturated fat, 2 g protein, 6 g carbohydrates, 2 g fiber, 162 mg sodium

MAKE IT A SALT SOLUTION MEAL
Serve with any Salt Solution meal with 250 calories or less.

Curried Edamame

Prep time: 5 minutes ⬡ **Cook time:** 8 minutes ⬡ **Total time:** 13 minutes ⬡ MAKES 4 SERVINGS

1 bag (1 pound) frozen, unshelled edamame

2 teaspoons olive oil

1 teaspoon dark sesame oil

1 teaspoon curry powder

½ teaspoon ground coriander

1 tablespoon chopped fresh cilantro

¼ teaspoon kosher or coarse sea salt

1. Bring a large pot of water to a boil over high heat. Add the edamame and cook until bright green, about 5 minutes, and drain.

2. Heat the olive and sesame oils in a large nonstick skillet over medium-high heat. Add the curry powder and coriander and cook, stirring, until fragrant, about 30 seconds. Add the edamame and cook, tossing, until hot and well coated, about 2 minutes. Remove from the heat and stir in the cilantro and salt. Transfer to a bowl and serve.

Per serving: 169 calories, 7 g fat, 0 g saturated fat, 12 g protein, 17 g carbohydrates, 12 g fiber, 146 mg sodium

MAKE IT A SALT SOLUTION MEAL
Serve with 3 ounces grilled chicken breast, ¼ cup fat-free Greek-style yogurt mixed with ¼ cup diced cucumber and 1 cup cubed watermelon (309 calories and 202 mg sodium total).

Italian Baked Fries

Prep time: 10 minutes ▷ **Cook time:** 45 minutes ▷ **Total time:** 55 minutes ▷ MAKES 4 SERVINGS

2½ teaspoons olive oil
 ½ teaspoon Italian seasoning
 ½ teaspoon garlic powder
 ½ teaspoon salt-free spice blend
 1 tablespoon Parmesan cheese

 ⅛ teaspoon salt
 ¼ teaspoon cracked black pepper
 2 large Yukon gold potatoes
  (12 ounces), scrubbed and cut
  lengthwise into ½"-thick strips

1. Preheat the oven to 350°F. Cover a baking sheet with foil and coat with cooking spray.

2. In a large resealable plastic bag, combine the oil, Italian seasoning, garlic powder, spice blend, cheese, salt, and pepper. Add the potatoes, seal the bag, and shake to coat. Spread on the prepared baking sheet.

3. Bake for 45 minutes, or until brown and crisp on both sides, turning halfway through the cooking time.

Per serving: 100 calories, 3 g fat, 1 g saturated fat, 2 g protein, 16 g carbohydrates, 1 g fiber, 104 mg sodium

MAKE IT A SALT SOLUTION MEAL
Serve with any Salt Solution meal with 200 calories or less.

Kale Crostini

Prep time: 10 minutes ⁓ **Cook time:** 10 minutes ⁓ **Total time:** 20 minutes ⁓ MAKES 4 SERVINGS

6 ounces crusty Italian bread, cut into 8 (½"-thick) slices

5 cloves garlic (1 whole, 4 thinly sliced)

2 tablespoons extra virgin olive oil

⅛ teaspoon crushed red-pepper flakes

1½ pounds kale, woody stems removed, thinly sliced

4 grape tomatoes, halved

1. Preheat the oven to 425°F.

2. Arrange the bread slices in a single layer on a large baking sheet. Lightly coat the slices with cooking spray. Bake until lightly golden and crisp, 5 to 6 minutes. Remove from the oven and rub with 1 whole garlic clove.

3. Meanwhile, heat the oil in a large nonstick skillet over medium heat. Add the sliced garlic and red-pepper flakes. Cook, stirring, until the garlic starts to soften, about 30 seconds. Add the kale, in batches if necessary, and cook until wilted and tender, about 3 to 4 minutes.

4. To serve, top the bread slices with the kale mixture, then top with a tomato half cut side down.

Per serving: 272 calories, 10 g fat, 2 g saturated fat, 10 g protein, 40 g carbohydrates, 5 g fiber, 323 mg sodium

Stir-Fried Kale with Roasted Soybeans

Prep time: 10 minutes ❧ **Cook time:** 7 minutes ❧ **Total time:** 17 minutes ❧ MAKES 4 SERVINGS

2 teaspoons olive oil

1 large clove garlic, finely chopped

1 teaspoon grated fresh ginger

¼ cup unsalted roasted soybeans

1 pound kale, stems removed, chopped into 1" pieces

1 tablespoon soy sauce

2 tablespoons low-sodium vegetable broth

1. In a large nonstick skillet, heat the oil over medium-high heat. Add the garlic and ginger and cook for 30 seconds. Reduce the heat to medium.

2. Add the soybeans and cook for 1 minute. Add the kale, soy sauce, and broth. Cook for about 5 minutes, or until the kale is wilted but not soggy.

Per serving: 132 calories, 6 g fat, 1g saturated fat, 8 g protein, 16 g carbohydrates, 4 g fiber, 294 mg sodium

MAKE IT A SALT SOLUTION MEAL
Serve with couscous pilaf (¼ cup whole wheat couscous, 1 tablespoon raisins, and 1 tablespoon pine nuts) and 1 small tangerine (323 calories and 299 mg sodium total).

SNACKS

Fresh Tomato Salsa with Homemade Tortilla Crisps

Prep time: 15 minutes ⁛ **Cook time:** 10 minutes ⁛ **Total time:** 30 minutes ⁛ MAKES 4 SERVINGS

¾ pound plum tomatoes, seeded and chopped

1 Hass avocado, peeled, pitted, and diced

1 cup no-salt-added pinto beans, rinsed and drained

1 jalapeño chile pepper, seeded and finely chopped (wear plastic gloves when handling)

1 cup fresh corn kernels

⅓ cup chopped red onion

3 tablespoons chopped fresh cilantro

1 tablespoon fresh lime juice

⅛ teaspoon + ¼ teaspoon salt

10 corn tortillas (6" diameter), cut into 6 wedges each

1. Preheat the oven to 425°F. Coat 2 large baking sheets with cooking spray.

2. In a medium bowl, combine the tomatoes, avocado, pinto beans, pepper, corn, onion, cilantro, lime juice, and ⅛ teaspoon of the salt. Set aside.

3. Arrange the tortilla wedges in a single layer on the baking sheets. Coat lightly with cooking spray, then sprinkle with the remaining ¼ teaspoon salt. Bake until lightly browned, about 10 minutes. Remove from the oven and allow to cool for 5 minutes. Transfer to a bowl and serve with the salsa.

Per serving: 294 calories, 8 g fat, 1 g saturated fat, 9 g protein, 51 g carbohydrates, 12 g fiber, 266 mg sodium

Spinach Hummus with Vegetable Dippers

Prep time: 15 minutes ⠶ **Total time:** 2 hours 15 minutes ⠶ MAKES 4 SERVINGS

1 can (15 ounces) no-salt-added
   chickpeas, rinsed and drained
4 cups baby spinach
1 cup fat-free plain yogurt
½ cup no-salt-added cannellini
   beans, rinsed and drained
1 clove garlic
3 tablespoons fresh lemon juice
2 teaspoons tahini

1½ teaspoons grated lemon zest
5 teaspoons extra virgin olive oil
1 red bell pepper, cut into 2" × ¼"
   strips
2 ribs celery, cut into 2" × ¼" strips
16 baby carrots
1 whole wheat pita, cut into
   12 wedges

1. In the bowl of a food processor, combine the chickpeas, spinach, yogurt, beans, garlic, lemon juice, tahini, and lemon zest, and puree. With the processor running, add the oil and process for 1 minute longer. Refrigerate for 2 hours before serving.

2. Serve with the bell pepper and celery strips, carrots, and pita wedges.

Per serving: 276 calories, 9 g fat, 1 g saturated fat, 12 g protein, 41 g carbohydrates, 9 g fiber, 296 mg sodium

Spinach Pesto Dip

Prep time: 10 minutes ⁑ **Total time:** 1 hour 10 minutes ⁑ MAKES 6 SERVINGS

1 package (10 ounces) frozen chopped spinach, thawed and squeezed dry

½ cup thinly sliced scallions

½ cup finely chopped yellow bell pepper

4 tablespoons pesto

½ cup fat-free plain yogurt

2 tablespoons reduced-fat sour cream

2 tablespoons reduced-fat mayonnaise

1 clove garlic, minced

6 whole wheat pitas (4" diameter), cut into 8 wedges each

1 cup grape tomatoes

3 ribs celery, cut into 2"-long sticks

3 medium carrots, cut into 2"-long sticks

2 cooked baby red potatoes (about 12 ounces), cut into wedges

In a medium bowl, combine the spinach, scallions, bell pepper, pesto, yogurt, sour cream, mayonnaise, and garlic. Cover and chill for at least 1 hour before serving. Serve with the pita wedges, tomatoes, celery and carrot sticks, and potatoes.

Per serving: 219 calories, 7 g fat, 2 g saturated fat, 9 g protein, 33 g carbohydrates, 6 g fiber, 321 mg sodium

MAKE IT A SALT SOLUTION MEAL
Serve with 1½ tablespoons unsalted almonds (290 calories and 353 mg sodium total).

Artichoke Dip Arrabbiata

Prep time: 6 minutes ⁝▸ **Cook time:** 34 minutes ⁝▸ **Total time:** 40 minutes ⁝▸ MAKES 6 SERVINGS

1 tablespoon olive oil
¾ cup chopped onion
¼ cup crumbled precooked bacon
1 container (15 ounces) fat-free ricotta cheese
1 can (14 ounces) artichoke hearts, rinsed, drained, and torn into chunks

½ cup canned unsalted petite-diced tomatoes, drained
½ teaspoon red-pepper flakes
2 tablespoons shredded Parmesan-Romano-Asiago cheese blend
4 whole wheat pitas (4" diameter), toasted and cut into 8 wedges each

1. Preheat the oven to 350°F.

2. In an 8" × 8" microwaveable baking dish, combine the oil, onion, and bacon. Cover with plastic wrap, leaving a small corner vent. Microwave on high power for 4 minutes, or until the onion is pale golden.

3. Add the ricotta cheese, artichokes, tomatoes, red-pepper flakes, and 1 tablespoon of the cheese blend. Stir to mix thoroughly.

4. Bake for 30 minutes, or until bubbling. Serve with the pita wedges.

Per serving: 176 calories, 5 g fat, 1 g saturated fat, 14 g protein, 21 g carbohydrates, 5 g fiber, 314 mg sodium

MAKE IT A SALT SOLUTION MEAL
Serve with 1 tangerine (270 calories and 232 mg sodium total).

Personal White Pizza

Prep time: 10 minutes ⁕ **Cook time:** 15 minutes ⁕ **Total time:** 25 minutes ⁕ MAKES 4

3 large cloves garlic, finely chopped
2 teaspoons canola oil
½ cup fat-free ricotta cheese
2 tablespoons ground flaxseed
2 tablespoons nonfat dry milk

4 whole wheat flour tortillas
(9–10" diameter)
3 tablespoons grated Parmesan
cheese
2 slices (¼ ounce each) reduced-fat
Swiss cheese, finely chopped

1. Preheat the oven to 375°F.

2. In a small microwaveable bowl, combine the garlic and oil. Cover with plastic wrap, leaving a corner vent. Microwave for 1 minute, or until sizzling. Remove and let stand for 5 minutes.

3. Add the ricotta, flaxseed, and dry milk to the garlic mixture. Stir until smooth.

4. Place the tortillas on 1 large or 2 smaller baking sheets. Spread the tortillas evenly with the ricotta mixture. Sprinkle the cheeses evenly over the tortillas.

5. Bake for 15 minutes, or until bubbly and golden.

Per serving: 193 calories, 8 g fat, 2 g saturated fat, 14 g protein, 25 g carbohydrates, 3 g fiber, 297 mg sodium

MAKE IT A SALT SOLUTION MEAL
Serve with 1 small banana (283 calories and 298 mg sodium total).

Sardines and White Beans

Prep time: 6 minutes ⁑ **Total time:** 6 minutes ⁑ MAKES 2 SERVINGS

1 can (3¾ ounces) low-sodium
    sardines
1½ cups chopped watercress
1 cup no-sodium-added canned
    white beans, drained

2 tablespoons low-fat creamy garlic
    dressing
1 teaspoon red wine vinegar

Cut the sardines crosswise into quarters in the can, then place in a bowl. Toss with the watercress, beans, dressing, and vinegar.

Per serving: 230 calories, 9 g fat, 4 g saturated fat, 15 g protein, 23 g carbohydrates, 6 g fiber, 101 mg sodium

MAKE IT A SALT SOLUTION MEAL
Serve with half a whole wheat roll (305 calories and 235 mg sodium total).

SWEETS AND DESSERTS

(Limit sweets and desserts to no more than one per day.)

Dried Fruit, Chocolate Chip, Pretzel, and Nut Mix

Prep time: 5 minutes ⊳ **Cook time:** 6 minutes ⊳ **Total time:** 11 minutes ⊳ MAKES 4 SERVINGS

2 ounces slivered almonds

1 cup dried apricots, chopped

½ cup raisins

2 ounces unsalted small pretzel twists

¼ cup semisweet chocolate chips

1. Heat a small nonstick skillet over medium heat. Add the almonds and cook, shaking the pan often, until toasted, about 6 minutes. Transfer to a bowl and cool for 5 minutes.

2. Add the apricots, raisins, pretzels, and chocolate chips to the bowl. Stir well and serve.

Per serving: 319 calories, 11 g fat, 3 g saturated fat, 6 g protein, 55 g carbohydrates, 6 g fiber, 48 mg sodium

Spiced Cereal and Nut Mix

Prep time: 10 minutes ⁞ᐅ **Cook time:** 26 minutes ⁞ᐅ **Total time:** 36 minutes ⁞ᐅ MAKES 6 SERVINGS

3 cups Total cereal

2 cups Corn Chex cereal

¼ cup sliced almonds

2 tablespoons olive oil

1 tablespoon maple syrup

2 teaspoons Worcestershire sauce

2 teaspoons ground cumin

1 teaspoon onion powder

⅛ teaspoon salt

¼ cup golden raisins

1. Preheat the oven to 350°F. Coat a large baking sheet with cooking spray.

2. In a large bowl, combine the cereals and almonds. Heat the oil in a small nonstick skillet over medium heat until warm. Stir in the maple syrup, Worcestershire sauce, cumin, onion powder, and salt. Cook for 30 seconds. Stir into the cereal mixture in 2 batches for better distribution. Pour onto the prepared baking sheet.

3. Place the baking sheet in the oven and reduce the temperature to 200°F. Bake for 25 minutes. Remove from the oven and stir in the raisins. Cool completely. Store in a zip-top resealable bag for up to 2 weeks.

Per serving: 202 calories, 7 g fat, 1 g saturated fat, 3 g protein, 33 g carbohydrates, 3 g fiber, 290 mg sodium

MAKE IT A SALT SOLUTION MEAL
Serve with 1 cup grapes (306 calories and 293 mg sodium total).

Curried Snack Mix with Dried Cherries

Prep time: 15 minutes ⁝⁘ **Cook time:** 50 minutes ⁝⁘ **Total time:** 1 hour 15 minutes
⁝⁘ MAKES 8 SERVINGS

3 whole wheat pitas (4" diameter), halved crosswise and thinly sliced

2 cups Wheat Chex cereal

1 cup minipretzels

4 ounces whole roasted almonds

1 tablespoon unsalted butter

½ tablespoon curry powder

½ tablespoon sugar

¾ teaspoon Worcestershire sauce

½ teaspoon garlic powder

¼ teaspoon paprika

¼ teaspoon ground coriander

⅛ teaspoon crushed red-pepper flakes

¾ cup dried cherries

1. Preheat the oven to 400°F. Coat a baking sheet with cooking spray. Spread the pita strips on the baking sheet and bake until crisp, about 7 to 8 minutes. Reduce the oven temperature to 200°F.

2. Remove from the oven, transfer to a bowl, and let cool for 5 minutes. Stir in the cereal, pretzels, and almonds.

3. In a small saucepan over medium heat, combine the butter, curry powder, sugar, Worcestershire sauce, garlic powder, paprika, coriander, and red-pepper flakes. Cook, stirring often, until the butter melts and the spices toast slightly, about 3 to 4 minutes. Stir into the cereal mixture and toss well to coat.

4. Pour the mixture onto a baking sheet and bake until crisp, 40 to 45 minutes. Remove from the oven, stir in the cherries, and cool completely before serving.

Per serving: 250 calories, 10 g fat, 2 g saturated fat, 7 g protein, 37 g carbohydrates, 6 g fiber, 294 mg sodium

MAKE IT A SALT SOLUTION MEAL
Serve with 1 small apple (305 calories and 295 mg sodium total).

Dried Apricot and Nut Biscotti

Prep time: 15 minutes ⁣ **Cook time:** 55 minutes ⁣ **Total time:** 1 hour 10 minutes
⁣ MAKES 10

2½ cups all-purpose flour
  1 cup sliced almonds
¾ cup dried apricots, chopped
½ cup nonfat dry milk
  2 teaspoons baking powder
  1 teaspoon ground ginger
½ teaspoon ground cinnamon

¾ cup sugar
  2 large eggs
⅓ cup orange juice with added
    calcium
½ teaspoon vanilla extract
¼ teaspoon almond extract

1. Preheat the oven to 350°F. Coat a baking sheet with cooking spray and set aside.

2. In the bowl of an electric mixer, combine the flour, almonds, apricots, dry milk, baking powder, ginger, and cinnamon. In a separate bowl, combine the sugar, eggs, orange juice, vanilla extract, and almond extract. Add the sugar mixture to the flour mixture and beat on low speed until well combined and a fairly dry dough forms. Press the dough into a ball and divide in half. On a lightly floured surface, use the palms of your hands to shape each half of the dough into a cylinder about 12" long × 1½" high × 1¾" wide. Transfer the dough to the prepared baking sheet and pat down the tops until the cylinders are about ¾" high and 2" wide.

3. Bake for 23 to 25 minutes, or until firm to the touch and a toothpick inserted into the dough comes out clean. Transfer the cookie logs to a cutting board and let cool for 10 minutes. With a serrated knife, cut the logs straight across into a total of fifty ¼"-thick slices. Arrange the cookies in a single layer on the baking sheet. Lower the oven temperature to 300°F. Bake for 15 minutes, turn the cookies, and bake for 15 minutes longer. Transfer the cookies to a wire rack. They will crisp as they cool.

Per serving: 291 calories, 6 g fat, 1 g saturated fat, 9 g protein, 52 g carbohydrates, 3 g fiber, 145 mg sodium

Pumpkin-Maple Cheesecake

Prep time: 15 minutes **Cook time:** 1 hour 10 minutes **Total time:** 5 hours 25 minutes
 MAKES 16 SERVINGS

3 packages (8 ounces each) fat-free cream cheese, at room temperature

²/₃ cup packed brown sugar

3 large eggs

1 can (15 ounces) pure pumpkin

½ cup low-fat maple or vanilla yogurt

2 tablespoons all-purpose flour

1½ teaspoons ground cinnamon

1 teaspoon ground ginger

1 teaspoon maple or rum flavoring

1 teaspoon vanilla extract

1 cup toasted pumpkin seeds

1. Preheat the oven to 350°F. Coat a 9" springform pan with cooking spray.

2. In the bowl of an electric mixer, beat together the cream cheese and brown sugar until smooth. Beat in the eggs one at a time. Blend in the pumpkin, yogurt, flour, cinnamon, ginger, maple or rum flavoring, and vanilla extract. Pour the filling into the prepared pan. Bake for 1 hour and 10 minutes.

3. Remove from the oven and run a knife around the sides to loosen. Let stand at room temperature for 30 minutes. Chill the cake, uncovered, until cold. Then cover with foil and chill for at least 4 hours (or up to 3 days).

4. When ready to serve, carefully remove the sides of the pan. Sprinkle each serving with 1 tablespoon of the pumpkin seeds.

Per serving: 189 calories, 7 g fat, 2 g saturated fat, 13 g protein, 19 g carbohydrates, 1 g fiber, 328 mg sodium

MAKE IT A SALT SOLUTION MEAL
Serve with 2 tablespoons pecans (275 calories and 328 mg sodium total).

Banana Nut Cake

Prep time: 10 minutes ⫶⫶ **Cook time:** 30 minutes ⫶⫶ **Total time:** 1 hour ⫶⫶ MAKES 12 SERVINGS

CAKE
- ²/₃ cup granulated sugar
- 2 ripe bananas, mashed
- 2 large eggs
- ²/₃ cup fat-free milk
- 2 tablespoons canola oil
- 1 teaspoon vanilla extract
- 1¾ cups all-purpose flour
- 2 teaspoons baking powder
- 1 teaspoon ground cinnamon
- ¼ teaspoon salt
- 1 cup Brazil nuts, chopped

GLAZE
- 1 cup confectioners' sugar
- 1 tablespoon fat-free milk
- 1 teaspoon vanilla extract

1. *To make the cake:* Preheat the oven to 350°F. Coat a 9" × 9" baking pan with cooking spray and lightly coat with flour.

2. In a large bowl, combine the granulated sugar, bananas, eggs, milk, oil, and vanilla extract, mixing well. In a separate bowl, combine the flour, baking powder, cinnamon, and salt. Add the flour mixture to the banana mixture and stir until just combined. Fold in the Brazil nuts. Pour the batter into the baking pan.

3. Bake for 28 to 30 minutes, or until a toothpick inserted in the center comes out clean. Cool in the pan for 10 minutes. Turn out of the pan onto a rack to cool completely.

4. *To make the glaze:* Meanwhile, in a small bowl, combine the confectioners' sugar, milk, and vanilla extract. Spread the glaze over the cake with a small spatula. Cut into 12 squares.

Per serving: 275 calories, 11 g fat, 2 g saturated fat, 6 g protein, 41 g carbohydrates, 2 g fiber, 148 mg sodium

Lemon-Buttermilk Bundt Cake

Prep time: 20 minutes ⋮➤ **Cook time:** 38 minutes ⋮➤ **Total time:** 1 hour 43 minutes
⋮➤ MAKES 14 SERVINGS

3 cups all-purpose flour
1½ cups sugar
2 teaspoons baking powder
½ teaspoon baking soda
¼ teaspoon salt
1 cup low-fat buttermilk
½ cup dry buttermilk
2 large eggs

6 tablespoons canola oil
⅓ cup fresh lemon juice
1 tablespoon grated lemon zest
4 medium bananas, sliced
2 cups strawberries, hulled and
 sliced
1 cup fresh blueberries

1. Preheat the oven to 350°F. Coat a 10" tube or Bundt pan with cooking spray and sprinkle lightly with flour to coat.

2. In the bowl of an electric mixer, combine the flour, 1 cup plus 6 tablespoons of the sugar, the baking powder, baking soda, and salt. Mix on low to combine. In a separate bowl, combine the buttermilk and dry buttermilk and mix well. Whisk in the eggs, oil, lemon juice, and lemon zest. Add the buttermilk mixture to the flour mixture and mix on low speed for 2 minutes, or until well combined. Pour into the prepared pan.

3. Bake in the center of the oven for 35 to 38 minutes, or until a toothpick inserted into the cake comes out clean. Cool in the pan on a wire rack for 15 minutes. Remove the cake from the pan and cool on the rack for 30 minutes before slicing.

4. Meanwhile, in a medium bowl, combine the bananas, strawberries, blueberries, and the remaining 2 tablespoons sugar. Serve with the sliced cake.

Per serving: 299 calories, 7 g fat, 1 g saturated fat, 6 g protein, 55 g carbohydrates, 2 g fiber, 204 mg sodium

Healthy Bread Pudding

Prep time: 8 minutes ⊳ **Cook time:** 40 minutes ⊳ **Total time:** 48 minutes ⊳ MAKES 6 SERVINGS

4 cups stale whole grain bread
(about 6–8 slices), cut into
½" cubes

1 cup fat-free half-and-half

1 cup fat-free milk

1 cup fresh or frozen blueberries

2 teaspoons grated orange zest

3 large eggs, beaten

2 egg whites, lightly beaten

⅓ cup brown sugar

1 teaspoon vanilla extract

¼ teaspoon ground allspice

1 tablespoon light butter, softened

1. Preheat the oven to 350°F. Coat an 8-cup baking dish with cooking spray. Place the bread cubes in the baking dish. Set aside.

2. In a large bowl, mix the half-and-half, milk, ½ cup of the blueberries, orange zest, eggs and egg whites, sugar, vanilla extract, and allspice. Stir until well mixed.

3. Pour the mixture over the bread cubes and stir just until coated. Top the pudding with the remaining ½ cup blueberries, and dot the bread with the softened butter. Bake uncovered for 40 minutes, or until the top is golden and the pudding is firm to the touch.

Per serving: 238 calories, 6 g fat, 2 g saturated fat, 11 g protein, 36 g carbohydrates, 3 g fiber, 278 mg sodium

MAKE IT A SALT SOLUTION MEAL
Serve with ½ cup fat-free milk (281 calories and 342 mg sodium total).

Caramel Flan

Prep time: 20 minutes ⁞⊱ **Cook time:** 20 minutes ⁞⊱ **Total time:** 40 minutes ⁞⊱ MAKES 6 SERVINGS

²/₃ cup sugar

1 tablespoon water

3 large eggs

1½ cups 1% milk

1½ teaspoons vanilla extract

2 cups mixed raspberries, blackberries, and sliced kiwifruit

1. Preheat the oven to 325°F. In a heavy medium skillet over medium-high heat, combine ⅓ cup of the sugar and the water. Heat until the sugar is melted and caramelized (golden in color), stirring often.

2. Carefully pour the caramelized sugar (it will be very hot) evenly into six 4-ounce ramekins or custard cups. Tilt the ramekins to coat the bottoms. Let stand for 10 minutes.

3. In a medium bowl, whisk the eggs and the remaining ⅓ cup sugar until well blended. Whisk in the milk and vanilla extract. Transfer the mixture to a large glass measuring cup or pitcher for easier handling. Pour evenly into the ramekins.

4. Place the ramekins in a baking pan just large enough to hold them without touching. Place the pan on the oven rack and pour hot water into the pan to a depth of ½".

5. Bake the flans for 20 to 25 minutes, or until a knife inserted near the center comes out clean. Carefully lift the ramekins from the hot water onto a wire rack. Serve warm or cool completely, cover, and refrigerate for up to 24 hours. Garnish with the fresh fruit.

Per serving: 252 calories, 5 g fat, 2 g saturated fat, 11 g protein, 40 g carbohydrates, 2 g fiber, 135 mg sodium

 MAKE IT A SALT SOLUTION MEAL
Serve with 1 tablespoon unsalted almonds (304 calories and 135 mg sodium total).

Cardamom Rice Pudding

Prep time: 5 minutes ⁂ **Cook time:** 1 hour ⁂ **Total time:** 1 hour 5 minutes ⁂ MAKES 4 SERVINGS

1¹⁄₃ cups cooked rice
2²⁄₃ cups 2% milk
  1 egg, beaten
  ¼ cup sugar

3 tablespoons coarsely ground
  almonds
1 teaspoon vanilla extract
½ teaspoon ground cinnamon
½ teaspoon ground cardamom

1. Preheat the oven to 350°F. Coat a medium round ceramic dish with cooking spray.

2. In a large bowl, combine the rice, milk, egg, sugar, almonds, vanilla extract, cinnamon, and cardamom. Spread evenly in the prepared dish.

3. Bake for 15 minutes. Stir to recombine. Repeat twice for a total cooking time of 45 minutes. Bake for an additional 10 to 15 minutes, or until the pudding reaches the desired consistency. Refrigerate.

Per serving: 237 calories, 5 g fat, 2 g saturated fat, 10 g protein, 37 g carbohydrates, 1 g fiber, 90 mg sodium

MAKE IT A SALT SOLUTION MEAL
Serve with 1 small banana (327 calories and 91 mg sodium total).

Tropical Fruit Salad

Prep time: 15 minutes ⋮⊳ **Total time:** 45 minutes ⋮⊳ MAKES 4 SERVINGS

1 mango, cut into ½" pieces
½ pineapple, cut into ½" pieces
   (about 3 cups)
3 bananas, halved lengthwise and
   cut crosswise into 1"-thick slices

1 Hass avocado, cut into 1" pieces
2 tablespoons fresh lime juice
2 tablespoons honey
1 tablespoon chopped fresh cilantro

In a large bowl, combine the mango, pineapple, bananas, avocado, lime juice, honey, and cilantro. Toss well. Let stand for 30 minutes before serving.

Per serving: 283 calories, 8 g fat, 1 g saturated fat, 3 g protein, 57 g carbohydrates, 8 g fiber, 7 mg sodium

Minted Melon Soup

8 cups cubed honeydew melon or cantaloupe	1 tablespoon honey
$\frac{1}{4}$ cup lemon or lime juice	$\frac{1}{8}$ teaspoon almond extract
8 fresh mint leaves	$\frac{1}{4}$ teaspoon ground nutmeg
	Pinch of salt

1. In a large food processor or blender, puree the melon or cantaloupe, juice, mint, honey, almond extract, nutmeg, and salt.

2. Refrigerate for at least 1 hour or up to 2 days.

Per serving: 143 calories, 1 g fat, 0 g saturated fat, 2 g protein, 37 g carbohydrates, 3 g fiber, 134 mg sodium

MAKE IT A SALT SOLUTION MEAL
Serve with 1 cup unsalted cottage cheese (306 calories and 160 mg sodium total).

Maple Strawberry Bananas Foster

Prep time: 5 minutes ❉ **Cook time:** 5 minutes ❉ **Total time:** 10 minutes ❉ MAKES 4 SERVINGS

1 tablespoon unsalted butter

3 medium bananas, sliced

1½ cups fresh strawberries, hulled
 and sliced

⅓ cup orange juice with calcium

¼ cup maple syrup

⅛ teaspoon ground cinnamon

2 cups fat-free vanilla frozen yogurt

1. Melt the butter in a large nonstick skillet over medium-high heat. Add the bananas and strawberries. Cook, stirring occasionally, until starting to soften, about 2 to 3 minutes. Stir in the orange juice, maple syrup, and cinnamon. Bring mixture to a boil, stirring occasionally, and cook until slightly thickened, about 2 minutes. Remove from the heat.

2. Scoop ½ cup of the frozen yogurt into each of 4 bowls. Top each with ½ cup fruit mixture and serve immediately.

Per serving: 278 calories, 4 g fat, 2 g saturated fat, 6 g protein, 59 g carbohydrates, 3 g fiber, 68 mg sodium

Easy Chocolate Pudding with Banana

Prep time: 5 minutes · **Cook time:** 8 minutes · **Total time:** 2 hours 13 minutes
· MAKES 4 SERVINGS

2 medium bananas

2 cups 1% milk

$\frac{1}{2}$ cup sugar

$\frac{1}{4}$ cup unsweetened cocoa powder

3 tablespoons cornstarch

$1\frac{1}{2}$ ounces semisweet chocolate, chopped

1 teaspoon vanilla extract

1. Slice 1 banana. Line the bottom of four 6-ounce ramekins or custard cups with the banana slices.

2. In a medium saucepan, whisk together the milk, sugar, cocoa powder, and cornstarch. Bring to a boil over medium heat, stirring constantly. Boil, stirring, for 1 minute, or until thickened. Remove from the heat and stir in the chocolate and vanilla extract until the chocolate melts and the pudding is smooth, about 45 seconds. Divide the pudding among the ramekins or custard cups. Press a piece of plastic wrap directly onto the pudding and chill for at least 2 hours.

3. Remove the plastic from the pudding. Slice the remaining banana, top each pudding with the slices, and serve.

Per serving: 281 calories, 4 g fat, 2 g saturated fat, 6 g protein, 60 g carbohydrates, 4 g fiber, 55 mg sodium

Strawberry Thick Shake

Prep time: 5 minutes ꞏ **Total time:** 5 minutes ꞏ MAKES 2 SERVINGS

2 cups strawberry low-fat ice cream
¾ cup very cold 1% milk
6 large strawberries, hulled

1 tablespoon vanilla syrup
2 ice cubes

In a blender, combine the ice cream, milk, strawberries, syrup, and ice cubes and process until smooth. Pour into 2 glasses and serve immediately.

Per serving: 283 calories, 4 g fat, 2 g saturated fat, 7 g protein, 52 g carbohydrates, 3 g fiber, 110 mg sodium

Soy Hot Chocolate

Prep time: 1 minute ⁞► **Cook time:** 2 minutes ⁞► **Total time:** 3 minutes ⁞► MAKES 1 SERVING

1 cup vanilla soymilk

2 teaspoons maple syrup

2 teaspoons unsweetened cocoa powder

4 miniature marshmallows

Pour the soymilk into a microwaveable mug and microwave for about 2 minutes. Before it begins to boil, add the maple syrup and cocoa powder. Mix until frothy. Add the marshmallows and serve.

Per serving: 152 calories, 4 g fat, 0 g saturated fat, 7 g protein, 23 g carbohydrates, 1 g fiber, 99 mg sodium

MAKE IT A SALT SOLUTION MEAL
Serve with 2 graham crackers (272 calories and 184 mg sodium total).

Sodium
SLEUTHING

Our food supply is loaded with salt. From the saltshaker on your dinner table, to the fast food you pick up on the go, to many of your favorite products in the grocery store, salt is everywhere. Before you start to panic, though, keep in mind that grocery shopping and preparing meals at home doesn't have to be complicated. With the simple sodium-sleuthing tips for grocery shopping and cooking provided in this chapter, you'll learn how to buy and prepare meals that are delicious, easy to put together, and still low in sodium.

The surest and simplest way to limit the salt in your food is to cook it yourself. When you choose the recipes and ingredients, you are also choosing how much salt you consume. Getting back to cooking basics and minimizing the role of processed and fast foods will do wonders for your health and your waistline. But while it would be great for your sodium levels if you prepared all your meals at home and completely eliminated processed foods, we know this isn't possible for most of us with our overscheduled lives. Since convenience is key to helping you stick with a low-salt diet, we'll also provide tips on which pack-aged foods are lowest in sodium and tricks on how best to incorporate some of them into your diet.

Keeping salt levels low even while eating some processed and restaurant foods should become even easier soon, as you will be seeing more low-sodium products in your grocery aisles and favorite fast-food chains. In April 2010, a report released by the Institute of Medicine recommended a new, coordinated approach to gradually reduce the sodium content in food, one requiring new government standards for acceptable levels.[1] In anticipation of the report, large food companies such as Kraft, Campbell's, General Mills, and PepsiCo all said they planned to take steps to reduce the sodium levels in their various prod-ucts.[2] Meanwhile, New York City's health department has called on restaurant chains and food producers to lower the amount of salt in their products by 25 percent over the next 5 years, spurring even more food companies, such as Starbucks and H. J. Heinz Co., to jump aboard the low-sodium train.[3, 4]

But there's no need to wait for new products to appear before you start making changes. By following the tips and tricks provided in this chapter and the next, you'll be on your way to developing low-sodium habits that will last a lifetime.

Supermarket Sodium Savvy

PREPARING A DELICIOUS LOW-SODIUM MEAL begins in the grocery store. This is where your sodium-sleuthing skills will come in handy the most, as supermarket aisles can be full of sodium minefields. Fortu-nately, there are lots of tricks you can use to avoid saboteurs of your new healthy habits.

First things first. Don't leave home without a list, as it's too easy to get sidetracked by unhealthy options without one. Include all the ingredients you'll need for your Salt Solution meals, including low-sodium staples. Don't forget the snacks and treats. Making a list will keep you on the low-sodium track and save you time. You also want to make sure you don't go shopping on an empty stomach. Nothing will make you lose your sodium savvy like a growling stomach, as suddenly all those high-fat, high-sodium products call your name.

Stock Up on Staples

Having a low-sodium-stocked kitchen is the first step to sticking to this lifestyle. There are many foods you can keep on hand that are good for you and have little salt, including flavor boosters and healthy snacks. These staples will become particularly important when unhealthy food cravings kick in or you're short on time, and will make it less tempting to turn to not-so-good-for-you options. So be sure to keep these staples on hand at all times.

PANTRY STAPLES

Dried herbs and spices (see "The Salt Solution Seasoning Guide" on page 204)

Low-sodium seasonings like Mrs. Dash and Spice Hunter

Flavored vinegars like sherry vinegar, red wine vinegar, champagne vinegar, and rice vinegar

Olive oil

Canned fruit (packed in its own juice or water, not heavy syrup)

Low-sodium or unsalted canned vegetables, including tomato products

Low-sodium or unsalted canned or dehydrated soups, broth, and bouillon

Whole grain and low-sodium bread

Whole grain pasta

Brown rice

Unsalted seeds and nuts, such as almonds and walnuts

Dried peas, beans, and lentils, including Salt Solution Stars such as white beans

Unsalted or low-salt canned peas, beans, and lentils, including Salt Solution Stars such as white beans

Roasted soybeans, a Salt Solution Star

Low-sodium canned fish, including Salt Solution Stars such as sardines

Low-sodium ready-to-eat cereals and oatmeal

Unsalted popcorn and pretzels

FRIDGE STAPLES

Fresh herbs (see "The Salt Solution Seasoning Guide" on page 204)

Onions

Fruits, including Salt Solution Stars such as bananas

Vegetables, including Salt Solution Stars such as beet greens, kale, spinach, and sweet potatoes

Fat-free or 1% milk and yogurt (all are Salt Solution Stars)

Soymilk (a Salt Solution Star)

Fat-free, low-fat, or reduced-fat cheeses with low sodium, such as ricotta, mozzarella, and Swiss

Fresh lean meats, poultry, and fish that haven't been seasoned or breaded

Lemon juice, lemons

Lime juice, limes

Eggs and egg substitutes

Salsas and other low-sodium condiments

Unsalted margarine or butter

Water

FREEZER STAPLES

Frozen fruit (no-sugar-added varieties)

Frozen lean cuts of meat, poultry, and fish that haven't been seasoned or breaded

Frozen vegetables (varieties without added butter, sauces, or seasoning), including Salt Solution Stars such as spinach and soybeans, or edamame

You may be surprised to notice that there are no low-salt or no-salt substitutes on the list. These products replace some or all of the sodium chloride (ordinary salt) with potassium chloride and/or lysine, and they're fine to use (though you should consult your doctor if you have diabetes, heart conditions, or kidney disease). But between the freshness of the ingredients and the combination of herbs and spices, you'll find that the Salt Solution meals are bursting with so much flavor that you won't need them. See Fight the Salt Assault on page 193 for recommended low-sodium brands and products, and "The Salt Solution Seasoning Guide" on page 204 for food preparation tips.

The Claim Game

With a full stomach and your list in hand, it's time to go shopping. Keep in mind that taste alone may not tell you which foods are high in sodium, so you must read food labels to get the full picture. You need to be careful, though. Food packaging these days can be loaded with confusing health claims. It can be overwhelming to figure out what they all mean, especially since a health claim doesn't guarantee that the food is actually good for you. The same goes for sodium claims.

To clear up the confusion, here's a rundown of sodium claims you'll find on packaged foods and what they mean. You want to grab foods with these FDA-regulated claims when you're out shopping.[5]

Sodium free or salt free: Less than 5 milligrams of sodium per serving

Very low sodium: 35 milligrams or less of sodium per serving

Low sodium: 140 milligrams or less of sodium per serving

Low-sodium meal: 140 milligrams or less of sodium per 3½ ounces (100 grams)

Other sodium-related claims compare the original version of the product with one lower in sodium. This is where things can get tricky, because if the original version is high in salt, the newer version may be better but still not good for you. When you see these claims, it's better to turn the package around and look at exactly how much sodium is in the food. Those numbers will give you the whole story. Here's a rundown of these comparative sodium claims.

Reduced or less sodium: At least 25 percent less sodium than the regular version

Food Label Know-How

Think of the Nutrition Facts labels found on most packaged and processed foods as road maps to your healthy and low-sodium destination. Use the label to compare the amount of sodium in products, choosing the one with less sodium as well as less saturated fat, fewer calories, and more fiber. With a little label know-how, you'll be able to determine in 10 seconds or less if a product gets a Salt Solution pass or fail. Use this 6-point plan to compare products and fill your cart (and home) with the best the store has to offer. After a few trips to the store, sodium-sleuthing labels will become automatic and easy—like riding a bike!

Soup A:
Split Pea Soup

Nutrition Facts

Serving Size 1 cup (248 g)
Servings Per Container 2

Amount Per Serving

Calories 100

	% Daily Value
Total Fat 0 g	0%
Saturated Fat 0 g	0%
Trans Fat 0 g	
Cholesterol 0 mg	0%
Sodium 330 mg	14%
Total Carbohydrates 19 g	6%
Fiber 6 g	24%
Sugars 4 g	
Protein 7 g	

Vitamin A 15%	Vitamin C 6%
Calcium 4%	Iron 8%

INGREDIENTS: (VEGAN) FILTERED WATER, ORGANIC GREEN SPLIT PEAS, ORGANIC ONIONS, ORGANIC CELERY, ORGANIC CARROTS, ORGANIC BASIL, SEA SALT, ORGANIC GARLIC, SPICES*, ORGANIC BLACK PEPPER. *100% PURE HERBS AND SPICES.

Soup B:
Split Pea Soup

Nutrition Facts

Serving Size 1 cup (244 g)
Servings Per Container 2

Amount Per Serving

Calories 160

	% Daily Value
Total Fat 2 g	3%
Saturated Fat 0.5 g	3%
Trans Fat 0 g	
Cholesterol 0 mg	0%
Sodium 690 mg	29%
Carbohydrates 28 g	9%
Fiber 4g	16%
Sugars 3g	
Protein 9g	

Vitamin A 2%	Vitamin C 0%
Calcium 2%	Iron 10%

INGREDIENTS: WATER, PEAS, SPLIT PEAS, CELERY. CONTAINS LESS THAN 2% OF BACON (PORK CURED WITH WATER, SALT, SUGAR, SODIUM PHOSPHATE, SODIUM ERYTHORBATE, SODIUM NITRITE), MODIFIED FOOD STARCH, SUGAR, SALT, POTASSIUM CHLORIDE, CORN PROTEIN (HYDROLYZED), MALTED BARLEY FLOUR, YEAST EXTRACT, SPICE, NATURAL FLAVOR.

❷ **❹** **❺** **❸** **❻** **❶**

1. INGREDIENTS: This is the first place to look on a label. Do you recognize what's listed, or is the product full of chemicals, preservatives, artificial sweeteners, hydrogenated fats, and unrecognizable ingredients? Do you see additives that contain sodium, such as sodium bicarbonate, sodium citrate, sodium chloride, and sodium nitrate/nitrite, and flavor boosters such as monosodium glutamate (MSG)? You want the foods you put in your cart (and in your body!) to be as clean as possible, so turn it over and investigate. If the product is full of ingredients you don't recognize, put it back on the shelf. Soup A, for example, lists *real* foods including onions, carrots, basil, and sea salt (yes, a little salt is okay). Soup B, however, contains not only peas, celery, and salt, but also ingredients like sodium phosphate, sodium erythorbate, sodium nitrite, and modified food starch. You shouldn't need a chemistry degree to decipher what's in your food. Soup A gets an ingredient thumbs-up, while Soup B gets a thumbs-down.

2. SERVING SIZE: If the ingredient list checks out, look at the serving size and the number of "servings per container." What looks like a single-serving package (a bag of chips from the deli, say) could actually contain two or more servings. In these examples, one serving of soup equals 1 cup, but there are actually two servings in the packages. If you ate the whole thing, you would double your sodium, calories, and everything else.

3. SODIUM: Follow the Salt Solution recommendations, and choose foods that fit within the guideline of about 300 milligrams of sodium per meal, or 1 milligram of sodium per calorie. You'll notice that Soup B, with 690 milligrams, would not fit in the Salt Solution plan. Soup A, with 330 milligrams, is a much better choice.

4. CALORIES: It's simple—if you eat too many calories, you'll gain weight. The calorie section should be the next part of the label you examine. Again, keep your Salt Solution guidelines of about 300 calories per meal in mind when selecting products. Soup A, with 100 calories per cup, and Soup B, with 160 calories per cup, would both fit within the Salt Solution calorie guidelines.

5. SATURATED AND TRANS FAT: Some fat is good for you, but you should limit the amount of saturated and trans fat (the "bad" fat that's been linked to heart disease) you consume. The Salt Solution limits saturated fat to no more than 3 grams per meal, and Soups A and B are within the limit.

6. FIBER: Fiber is a type of carbohydrate that your body can't digest, which means that it fills you up without adding extra calories. Salt Solution

(continued)

meals have at least 3 grams of fiber, but the more fiber, the better. Soup B, with 4 grams of fiber, is a good choice, but Soup A, with 6 grams (and much less sodium and whole ingredients instead of processed ones!), is much better.

Considering all points, Soup A is the clear Salt Solution winner. It's made with healthful whole ingredients and it's low in sodium, calories, and saturated fat, but full of filling fiber. Also, Soup A is higher in vitamins A and C, as well as calcium, because it's made with nutrient-rich vegetables.

Lite or light in sodium: 50 percent less sodium than the regular version

Unsalted or no salt added: No salt added to the product during processing (not a sodium-free food, as the product still contains the sodium that's a natural part of the food itself)

Other claims can also give you a clue about sodium levels. The Food and Drug Administration and the Department of Agriculture state that a food that has the claim "healthy" must not have more than 80 milligrams of sodium per reference amount. (The reference amount is the amount of food customarily eaten at one time, as set by the FDA; serving sizes listed on food labels must be close to these reference amounts.) "Meal type" products such as frozen dinners must not exceed 600 milligrams of sodium per serving size.[6]

These health claims can help you zero in on low-sodium products, but they still don't give you all the information you need to determine if a food will fit into the Salt Solution eating plan. First, even if a food is comparatively light in sodium, it may still have too much for you. Second, if a food is low in sodium but high in unhealthy saturated fats or added sugar, you will still gain weight. To get the full picture, you need to take a look at the Nutrition Facts label.

Beyond the Labels

What about foods without Nutrition Facts labels? Since you know by now that you want to eat fresh, whole foods (which tend not to come with labels), you might think that any foods without a label are a good bet. And, in fact, many of them are. At the grocery store and the salad bar, toss in plenty of fresh veggies and fruit. Fresh meat, poultry, and seafood are naturally low in sodium, but it's a good idea to find out more about calories and saturated fat before you make your purchases. Many supermarkets post nutrition information on posters or in brochures in the store, or you can check out the USDA nutrient database to get information on different foods at www.nal.usda.gov/fnic/foodcomp/search/. Congress is now considering legislation that would require nutrition labels on all raw meat and poultry products.

Where you want to be wary of foods without nutrition labels, however, is in the deli and salad bar sections of your supermarket. A good rule of thumb is to walk away from most of these prepared foods—salads packed with salty (and fattening) mayonnaise and other condiments, high-sodium soups, and cheese-covered pasta dishes. Even healthy-sounding grilled chicken and other meats normally found in salad bars are frequently salted before or after cooking, so go easy.

Fight the Salt Assault

SINCE YOU WANT YOUR EATING PLAN focused on mostly fresh and unprocessed foods, it's best to stick to the perimeter of the grocery store, where you'll find fresh produce, low-fat dairy products, and lean meats, poultry, and fish. The center aisles tend to be filled with processed foods, which you want to keep to a minimum.

But since we know there are going to be days when you're racing to get dinner on the table in the half hour between your daughter's soccer practice and your son's band rehearsal, we don't expect you to forgo the convenience of packaged foods altogether. And though processed and packaged foods can be high-salt traps, they're not all created equal. Some are definite sodium red flags and should be avoided or eaten in very small quantities. These include many canned foods, prepared mixes, and frozen dinners. (See "Top 10 Seriously Salty Foods in the Grocery Store" on page 210 for the list.)

But even within these categories, there are some brands and foods that tend to be lower in sodium than others. You can use your new label-reading skills to identify them, of course, but to make it even easier for you, we've compiled the following guide to the best low-sodium picks in the grocery store aisles. As you start to pay attention to the brands in your supermarket, you're sure to find even more low-salt options for each component of your Salt Solution meals. If you can't find the following brands or products in your grocery store, simply ask your store manager to order them. Most are more than happy to stock their shelves with requested items. Also consider ordering products online; we've provided Web sites for each brand when possible.

Protein

Meat and Poultry

Fresh meat is lower in sodium than processed meats such as cold cuts, hot dogs, sausage, and ham. In fact, usually smoked, cured, salted, or canned meat or poultry means high salt (see lunchmeat picks below). So go for fresh or frozen lean meats and poultry instead that haven't been injected with a sodium-containing solution. Many food manufacturers "enhance" meat by injecting it with a salt solution broth to keep it moist and improve its flavor. Check the ingredient list for sodium or salt, and check the product label for statements such as "self-basting" or "percent solution" or "broth," all terms that indicate that salt may have been added.

Lunchmeat

Whether your weakness is sliced turkey or roast beef, lunchmeats can be a time-saver. However, most brands and types are packed with salt. Although it may be challenging to find lower-salt options in the grocery store, the good news is that they do exist. Here are some you can try.

Boar's Head Oven-Roasted Choice Top Round, no salt added (www. boarshead.com/)

Dietz & Watson No Salt Added Breast of Turkey (www.dietzandwatson.net/)

Applegate Farms No Salt Turkey Breast (www.applegatefarms.com/)

Sardines, Tuna, and Salmon

All fish are loaded with heart-healthy omega-3 fats, including canned fish such as sardines, a Salt Solution Star. Canned fish is a fast way to get a dose of these good-for-you fats, but many brands pack a lot of salt into the can along with the fish. To avoid a high dose of sodium with your canned fish, seek out lower-salt options in these brands.

Roland Skinless & Boneless Sardines

StarKist Tuna (www.starkist.com/)

Bumble Bee Tuna (www.bumblebee.com/)

Chicken of the Sea Tuna (http://chickenofthesea.com/)

Crown Prince Natural Alaskan Pink Salmon (www.crownprince.com/)

Beans

When you're in a protein pinch, canned beans can be a major time-saver. Just add them to chili or your favorite salad and you have instant protein and fiber in your meal. The problem is that many companies add salt during the canning process, upping the sodium content. Try these brands for healthier options.

Eden Organic Plain Beans, Refried Beans, and Organic Seasoned Beans (www.edenfoods.com/)

Amy's Light in Sodium Organic Refried Beans (www.amys.com/)

Goya Low Sodium Beans (www.goya.com/)

Kuner's No Salt Added Beans (www.faribaultfoods.com/)

Baking in the Salt

Salt can lurk in the most surprising places, including baking powder and baking soda. The tiny bit you add to help your muffins rise adds sodium to your diet. That's why many baked goods are surprisingly high in sodium. Sodium content varies by brand, but most baking powders contain about 120 milligrams of sodium per ¼ teaspoon, and baking sodas have about 300 milligrams per ¼ teaspoon. If you bake frequently, switch to sodium-free baking powder and baking soda to cut this hidden salt.

Dairy

Cheese

A sprinkling of cheese makes most meals taste even better. The bad news is that many kinds of cheese, such as feta and Cheddar, are loaded with salt. And though many soft cheeses, like cream cheese and cottage cheese, are lower in fat and calories, they're also high in salt. Sticking with lower-salt cheeses, like ricotta and Swiss, can help decrease your salt intake, and so can choosing options in these brands.

Sargento (www.sargento.com/)

Alpine Lace (www.alpinelace.com/)

Heluva Good (www.heluvagood.com/)

Boar's Head (www.boarshead.com/)

Organic Valley (www.boarshead.com/)

Produce

Fruits and Veggies

Load up on fresh fruits and veggies—not only are they good for you, but most options are naturally low in sodium. Usually the more deeply colored the better, as these fruits and veggies tend to be higher in vitamins and minerals. When fresh produce isn't available, choose frozen or canned vegetables and fruits in water without added sugars, salt, and saturated and trans fats. Make sure frozen veggies don't have any added sauces or seasonings. Try these tasty picks.

(continued on page 200)

Understanding Organic

Green is the way to go these days, and food is no exception. Many people are turning to more ecofriendly organic options. Organic foods are produced without synthetic fertilizers, conventional pesticides, genetic engineering, irradiation, or sewage sludge. Organic animal products, such as meat and dairy, come from animals that are not given antibiotics or growth hormones.[7] The good news is that it's easy to pick out organic products at the grocery store. The U.S. Department of Agriculture has a certification program that's made it simple. Foods that meet their strict standards have a USDA Organic label, so look out for it the next time you're shopping. You may also notice that some packaged foods say "Made with Organic Ingredients." This means they contain at least 70 percent organic ingredients.[8]

Keep in mind, though, that some farmers who use organic methods don't pursue USDA certification. So don't hesitate to ask about farming methods if you're at a farmers' market or if you're thinking about joining a CSA. CSAs are community-supported agriculture programs for food distribution that usually consist of weekly delivery or pickup of vegetables, fruit, meat, and dairy from local farmers and ranchers. Join a CSA in your area and you'll not only support local agriculture, you'll also receive delicious and healthy unprocessed and naturally low-sodium food all season long! (To find a CSA in your area, check www.localharvest. org/csa/.)

Now the bad news. While organic products are good for the environment, they aren't always good for you. Organic doesn't automatically equal low sodium—or low sugar, fat, or calories for that matter—and as many organic foods, especially processed and packaged ones, are very high in salt. One serving of Amy's canned Organic Black Bean

Chili, for example, has 680 milligrams of sodium, 28 percent of your daily recommended intake.[9] Remember, too, that a high-salt product doesn't suddenly transform into a low-sodium choice just because it's organic. Heinz's organic and classic ketchup both have the same amount of sodium: 190 milligrams per tablespoon.[10] So be sure to read the food labels of all products carefully, even organic ones, to confirm that they're low in sodium and healthy. When you find a healthy option that fits into the Salt Solution lifestyle, go for the organic version if it exists. Since fresh fruits and veggies are low in sodium, the organic option is always a safe bet.

If eating organic all the time is too much for your wallet or if it's hard to find these foods in your area, don't despair. The key is to be selective about your purchases. If you're looking for a little guidance, the Environmental Working Group (EWG), an advocacy group for public health and environmental issues, suggests that consumers focus on buying organic alternatives for the 12 fruits and vegetables with the highest pesticide levels; they call these the dirty dozen.[11] So try to go for organics when possible for these foods (ranked in descending order beginning with those with the most pesticides).

CELERY

PEACHES

STRAWBERRIES

APPLES

BLUEBERRIES

NECTARINES

BELL PEPPERS

SPINACH

CHERRIES

KALE/COLLARD GREENS

POTATOES

GRAPES (IMPORTED)

Birds Eye Frozen Vegetables (look for "No Salt Added" varieties) (www. birdseyefoods.com/)

Green Giant Frozen Vegetables (look for "No Salt Added" varieties) (www. greengiantfresh.com/)

Del Monte Canned Fruit (look for "No Salt Added" varieties) (www. delmonte.com/)

Grains

Breads

Bread. It's hard to stay away from the carb-y goodness of it. We often crave toast in the morning, and sandwiches are a quick lunch option. But breads, like cereals, are often high in salt. Search out low-sodium options from these brands when the carb craving hits.

Manna Bread (www.naturespath.com/)

Food for Life (www.foodforlife.com/)

Pepperidge Farm (www.pepperidgefarm.com/)

Rice Mixes

There are few things simpler than boiling some water and adding a rice mix. It's flavorful, fast, and filling. These mixes are often loaded with high-salt seasonings, though, even before you get the chance to add your own salt. Low-sodium options may be trickier to find, but they do exist. These brands have products that fit into the Salt Solution eating plan.

Seeds of Change (www.seedsofchange.com/)

Goya (www.goya.com/)

Kashi (www.kashi.com/)

Eden Organic Canned Rice and Beans (www.edenfoods.com/)

Cereals

Breakfast is a must to start your day off on the right foot. Cereal is a quick choice for days when you're on the go; just be careful about what kind you eat. Many cereals are high in sodium, often even ones that contain other good stuff such as fiber. So get used to reading labels before buying your morning pick-me-up. Look for low-sodium varieties from these brands to get you started.

Kashi (www.kashi.com/)

Bear Naked (www.bearnaked.com/)

Arrowhead Mills (www.arrowheadmills.com/)

Health Valley (www.healthvalley.com/)

Post (for example, Shredded Wheat) (www.postcereals.com/)

Crackers and Chips

Having a snack attack? Don't fret, not all snack options will put your sodium level through the roof. Although it's true that you should steer clear of many snack-type foods, crackers are often a safe bet. Many brands, even big ones, make low-salt or no-salt cracker options. Believe it or not, there are also unsalted potato chips. Though these nutrient-poor snacks should be considered a once-in-a-while splurge, here are some brands to get you started.

Dare Breton Crackers (http://usa.darefoods.com/)

Wasa Crispbread (www.wasa-usa.com/)

Kettle Brand Unsalted Potato Chips (http://kettlefoods.com/)

Terra Au Naturel Unsalted Potato Chips (www.terrachips.com/)

Fat

Fats, like oils, are naturally low in sodium. But when selecting butter or margarine, make sure to choose unsalted varieties; salted butter and margarine can have almost 100 milligrams of salt per tablespoon! Also look for unsalted nuts, seeds, and nut butters.

Meals

Soups and Chili

Soups and chili are great comfort food, hitting the spot on cold days. They can also be high in protein and other nutrients. Unfortunately, these canned foods are also often high in salt. Here are some low-sodium brands that have choices you can stick with.

Amy's Light in Sodium Soups and Chili (www.amys.com/)

Campbell's Low Sodium Soups and Broth (www.campbellsoup.com/)

Progresso Reduced Sodium Soups (www.progressofoods.com/)

Health Valley No Salt Added Soups and Chili (www.healthvalley.com/)

Imagine Light in Sodium Soups (www.imaginefoods.com/)

Frozen Dinners

It's hard to avoid frozen meals, especially with our hectic lives. You just pop one into the microwave and voila! Instant meal. The problem is that most frozen meals are loaded with salt. Luckily, there are some good choices. For example, some of the flavors in the brands below are lower-sodium options.

Amy's Light in Sodium Meals (www.amys.com/)

Celentano Vegetarian Selects

Ethnic Gourmet Meals (www.ethnicgourmet.com/)

Kashi Frozen Entrees (http://kashi.com/)

Lean Cuisine (for example, Glazed Chicken) (www.leancuisine.com/)

Bars

When you're on the go, nothing hits the spot like a nutrition bar. They're easy to carry in your bag and are often chock-full of good stuff like protein and vitamins. Just make sure you don't end up with the bars that are also chockful of salt. These brands offer safe low-salt bets.

LUNA (www.lunabar.com/)

Lärabar (www.larabar.com/)

CLIF (www.clifbar.com/)

KIND (http://kindsnacks.com/)

The Salt Solution Seasoning Guide

Who needs salt when you have fresh herbs and spices? These seasonings can take any dish from just okay to fabulous! They boost flavor without adding sodium, calories, or fat. Use these no-calorie, no-sodium suggestions to add flavor and seasoning to your Salt Solution meals and/or recipes. We've highlighted those we think pair especially well with the Salt Solution Stars (listed in bold below), but feel free to experiment for yourself with these herbs and spices.

ALLSPICE: Allspice is used in Jamaican jerk seasonings and many soups, stews, and curries. It's pungent and fragrant and used in both savory and sweet foods. Try it in a **white bean** stew, with **sweet potatoes,** or in baked goods.

BASIL: Great in salsas, tomato sauce, and pesto. Use as a flavor boost in salads, on sandwiches, and in soups (especially tomato, **white bean,** and minestrone). Great with green vegetables like **beet greens, kale, spinach,** broccoli, and peas.

CHILI POWDER: Add chili powder to chili, of course, but also to any Mexican or Tex-Mex dish for a rich and spicy flavor.

CHIVES: Chives have a slight onion flavor and are good to add to beef and potato dishes. They should be added close to the end of cooking to get the best flavor.

CILANTRO: A key component of Latin American, Middle Eastern, and Southeast Asian cuisine, this pungent herb is the perfect finish to salsas and bean salads, and pairs excellently with citrus. Cilantro is great with poultry and seafood dishes, or as a sprinkle to brighten up the flavor of any meal.

CINNAMON: You know that cinnamon is delicious in baked goods. But you can also use it in savory dishes. Try cinnamon sprinkled on **sweet potatoes** and winter squashes or in chicken soups and stews.

CURRY POWDER: Curry powder is a blend of up to 20 different herbs and spices, including cardamom, cinnamon, coriander, nutmeg, and pepper. Use it to flavor soups and stews, or to add a kick to the following Salt Solution stars: **halibut, sardines, soybeans, spinach, kale,** and **beet greens.** Mix with **yogurt** for a quick marinade or as a topper for Asian dishes.

DILL: Great paired with smoked and fresh fish (like **halibut** and **sardines**), in salads, and with cabbage, green beans, beets, and **beet greens.** Dill can be added to potatoes, meat dishes, and stews.

GARLIC: Like pepper, you can add garlic to nearly everything for a salt-free flavor punch.

GINGER: Ginger provides a sweet and spicy note to many foods, and you can use it fresh or dried. Fresh ginger looks like a knobby root. Peel and grate it into your recipes. Dried ginger is usually ground. Whatever type you use, ginger is perfect in Asian, North African, Indian, and Caribbean cuisines.

MINT: Refreshing and versatile, mint can be used on lamb, in grain salads, infused into hot or iced tea, and added to lemonade. Great when added to fruit salad.

NUTMEG (and other spices such as ginger and cloves): These sweet-spicy seasonings go very well with **sweet potatoes** and all forms of winter squash. **Spinach,** carrots, asparagus, and green beans also pair well with nutmeg.

OREGANO: A staple of both Greek and Italian cooking, oregano can be used in marinara and other tomato-based sauces, on pizza, or mixed with lemon juice and olive oil to serve over grilled or roasted fish fillets (like **halibut**). Oregano adds depth to soups, especially **white bean** and vegetable soups.

PAPRIKA: Paprika has a sweet and smoky flavor that's perfect for many dishes, including barbecue and chili, and the cuisines of India, Morocco, Europe, and the Middle East.

PARSLEY: Often relegated to garnish duty, this overlooked herb is a key component for soups and stocks. A sprinkling over salads or grilled fish (like **halibut**) adds a light, fresh taste. It is a key component of tabbouleh and is great with grains, corn, and peas.

PEPPER: Try pepper on everything! Freshly ground is the most flavorful. Use it before, during, and after cooking to add a punch of flavor.

ROSEMARY: The herb of romance pairs wonderfully with meats, poultry, and fish (like **halibut**), especially when roasting. Also excellent in savory baked items such as bread and pizza. Use in marinades, or simply rub on roasts before cooking. Use sparingly as it can overwhelm.

SAGE: Excellent in stuffing, on poultry, and with veal. Sage is also delicious on pastas and in starchy bean dishes, like those made with **white beans.**

TARRAGON: The licorice flavor found in tarragon melds nicely with fish (like **halibut**) and chicken, as well as in salad dressings, veal recipes, and egg dishes. It's also good with green vegetables like **kale, spinach,** asparagus, broccoli, green beans, and peas. Tarragon can over-whelm a dish, so use it in moderation.

THYME: A great addition to mari-nades for fish (like **halibut**), poultry, and meat. Thyme has a strong flavor, so be sure to add it at the beginning of cooking to help mellow its flavor. A must for soups, stews, chili, and roasts.

Condiments, Sauces, and Dressings

Condiments

Condiments can be a killer when it comes to sodium. Eating just a little can rack up a lot of milligrams of salt. One tablespoon of ketchup, for instance, has 167 milligrams of sodium. Sauces such as teriyaki (690 milligrams of sodium per tablespoon) and soy sauce (up to 1,000 milligrams of sodium per tablespoon) are also high-sodium offenders.[12] So use condiments sparingly on your meals or better yet skip them altogether. If you just can't give up condiments, though, try these brands for lower-sodium options or make your own (see page 208).

Heinz No Salt Tomato Ketchup (www.heinz.com/)

Hunt's Tomato Ketchup, No Salt Added (www.hunts.com/)

Westbrae Natural (ketchup and mustard) (www.westbrae.com/)

Annie's Naturals (mustard) (www.anniesnaturals.com/)

B&G (relish) (www.bgfoods.com/)

Cascadian Farm (relish) (www.cascadianfarm.com/)

Spectrum (mayonnaise) (www.spectrumorganics.com/)

Kraft (mayonnaise) (www.kraftfoodscompany.com)

Boar's Head (mustard and horseradish) (www.boarshead.com/)

Pasta Sauces

If you don't have time to whip up a tomato sauce for your pasta, the jarred variety is a close second best. However, jarred and canned tomato products tend to be loaded with salt, and they're a definite red flag when trying to pinpoint high-salt foods in the supermarket. There are some companies, though, that make low-sodium pasta sauces. Here are some examples.

Amy's (www.amys.com/)

Eden Organic (www.edenfoods.com/)

Walnut Acres (www.walnutacres.com/)

Salad Dressings

The best salad dressing is plain old oil and vinegar. It's simple and delicious. You can also easily whip up a few homemade dressings to keep on hand (see page 208 for a few ideas). For days when that just won't cut it for your taste buds or you're really short on time, bottled dressings can come in handy. Keep in mind, however, that these premade dressings are often packed with artificial flavorings and a lot of salt. So stick with options from brands like the ones listed here.

Matsos Greek Dressing (www.matsosgreekdressing.com/)

Annie's Naturals (www.anniesnaturals.com/)

Wild Thymes Salad Refreshers (www.wildthymes.com/)

Salt Solution Easy Sauces and Condiments

TOMATO SAUCE: Sauté 3 cloves minced garlic, 1/2 cup chopped onion, and 1 teaspoon dried basil in 1 tablespoon extra-virgin olive oil until softened. Add 1 can (28 ounces) no-salt-added crushed tomatoes and 1 can (6 ounces) no-salt-added tomato paste. Cook, stirring occasionally, until thickened. Stir in 1/4 teaspoon salt and 1/4 teaspoon black pepper. (71 calories and 110 mg sodium per 1/2 cup)

TARTAR SAUCE: In a small bowl, combine 2 tablespoons sweet pickle relish, 1 tablespoon minced onion, and 1 cup fat-free mayonnaise. Mix well. (14 calories and 136 mg sodium per tablespoon)

SALSA: In a small bowl, combine 4 seeded and chopped plum tomatoes, 1/2 finely chopped red onion, 1 minced jalapeño chile pepper, 2 tablespoons fresh lime juice, 2 tablespoons chopped fresh cilantro, and 1/8 teaspoon salt. (22 calories and 77 mg sodium per 1/2 cup)

DRESSING: In a small bowl, whisk together 2 tablespoons minced shallots, 1 tablespoon white wine vinegar, 1/4 teaspoon Dijon mustard, 1/4 cup fat-free plain yogurt, 1/8 teaspoon salt, and 1/8 teaspoon black pepper. Add 2 tablespoons olive oil and whisk well. (38 calories and 46 mg sodium per tablespoon)

CITRUS DRESSING: In a small bowl, whisk together 1/4 cup orange juice, 1 tablespoon lime juice, 1 tablespoon honey, 1 teaspoon orange zest, 1 teaspoon lime zest, 1/8 teaspoon salt, and 1/8 teaspoon pepper. Add 2 tablespoons olive oil and 2 tablespoons chopped fresh cilantro and whisk well. (59 calories and 49 mg sodium per tablespoon)

PEAR-APRICOT RELISH: In a small bowl, combine 1 peeled, chopped ripe Bartlett pear, 1/4 cup chopped dried apricots, 1/4 cup finely chopped onion, 2 tablespoons cider vinegar, 1 tablespoon sugar, 1 tablespoon chopped fresh mint, and 1/8 teaspoon salt. (35 calories and 49 mg sodium per 1/4 cup)

LEMON-BASIL MAYO: In a small bowl, combine 1 cup fat-free mayonnaise, 2 tablespoons fresh lemon juice, 1 tablespoon lemon zest, and 3 tablespoons chopped fresh basil. Mix well and refrigerate for at least 1 hour before using. (14 calories and 126 mg sodium per tablespoon)

Crafty in the Kitchen

ONCE YOU'VE LUGGED THOSE GROCERIES home, there's a lot you can do in the kitchen to keep the sodium content of your meals low. Remember, when you prepare the food, you have control over the amount of sodium that goes into it. To maximize this control, you're better off starting out with a dish that's almost sodium free and adding flavor instead of beginning with sodium-laden meals. Your health and waistline aren't impacted just by the salt in your meals; fat and calories make an impact too. Some cooking techniques are healthier than others. It's best to grill, broil, poach, roast, or stir-fry your foods instead of frying them if you want to lower the fat and calories in your meals.

Consider these tricks to boost the flavor and healthiness of your meals while minimizing the salt.

Rinse It Out: Since canned foods such as tuna, beans, and vegetables are typically loaded with salt, it's best to thoroughly rinse these before cooking to wash away excess salt.

Forget the Salt: You can simply leave out the salt in many recipes, including casseroles, stews, and other main dishes, without making a difference in the flavor. Cook rice, pasta, and hot cereals without salt. Baked goods are generally an exception, though, since leaving out the salt could affect the texture and taste.

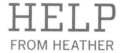

HELP
FROM HEATHER

What's the easiest way to save time and slash sodium?

Do what I do—load up on leftovers! Preparing food takes time, so why not make life easier for yourself? Try cooking low-sodium meals in bulk in the evening and then take the leftovers to work the next day. You'll save time and also be less tempted to turn to sodium-laden foods when your lunch cravings hit. You can also freeze leftovers so they're ready to go whenever hunger hits in the future.

Experiment with Unsalty Flavorings: Using fresh and dried herbs (see "The Salt Solution Seasoning Guide" on page 204), fresh pepper, low-sodium spices, flavored vinegars, garlic or garlic powder, and onions are all great ways to add flavor to your meals with minimal salt and fat. You can also try using fresh ginger, lemons, limes, or sodium-free bouillon. The flavor possibilities are endless, so be sure to experiment. To encourage you even further, consider keeping a spice mill or garlic press on hand instead of a saltshaker.

Dress It Up Simply: Sauces and salad dressings tend to be high in sodium. Instead of salad dressings, try using olive oil and vinegar or lemon juice on your leafy greens. For veggies, you can try herbs, spices, or lemon juice instead of heavy sauces. Be sure to limit the use of sodium-laden condiments, such as soy sauce, sauces, dips, ketchup, mustard, and relish. You can also prepare

Top 10 Seriously Salty Foods in the Grocery Store

1. FROZEN TV DINNERS = 4,000–4,500 milligrams per meal

2. FROZEN PIZZA = 1,000–1,200 milligrams per serving

3. PRETZEL RODS = 1,000–1,200 milligrams per serving

4. CANNED CHILI = 1000–1,200 milligrams per serving

5. LUNCHMEAT = 800–1,200 milligrams per serving

6. CANNED SOUP = 750–1,000 milligrams per serving

7. PACKAGED MACARONI AND CHEESE = 700–950 milligrams per serving

8. FLOUR TORTILLA = 550–650 milligrams per tortilla

9. CANNED VEGETABLES = 250–400 milligrams per serving

10. BREAKFAST CEREAL = 250–350 milligrams per serving

Note: We have listed the top of the sodium range for the above products.

your own version of condiments and other foods that tend to be high in salt, such as a simple tomato sauce for pasta and reduced-sodium soups. When you cook it, you control the salt. Check out the quick, everyday recipes on page 208. You can even take a stab at making salt-free bread or pizza dough. If you're nervous about making breads by hand, a bread machine is an easy alternative.

Doctor Prepared Meals: Add salt-free vegetables, beans, or grains to higher-sodium takeout or packaged foods. You'll cut the salt (by decreasing the sodium proportionately) and you'll increase fiber, potassium, and other nutrients. Some ideas: Mix half your favorite cereal with half of a sodium-free choice, such as puffed wheat. Add steamed or sautéed veggies such as broccoli or asparagus to your Chinese take-out dish. You can also try adding salt-free beans, lentils, or grains to these meals or to prepared mixes, such as flavored rices or ethnic food.

Are you ready to start living the Salt Solution way? Don't worry. It may seem daunting at first, but with our help you'll be able to handle any situation, including eating out, parties, and stressful times. Soon you'll start to automatically choose lower-sodium choices—and you'll start noticing changes in your waistline!

Salt Solution Success Story

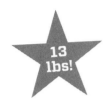

Beth Vorosmarti

Age: 47

Pounds Lost: 13

Inches Lost: 6¾ overall

BETH, A 47-YEAR-OLD HOMEMAKER AND ARTIST, used to be relatively fit, but she started struggling with her weight after her children were born. She stopped exercising regularly and the pounds started to pack on. Other programs didn't work, and then Beth found the Salt Solution. Beth appreciates that she doesn't have to cook different food for her family while she's following the Salt Solution program. With other diet programs she tried, she found herself buying expensive meal and snack replacements. "I think about the message I am sending to my kids that you have to eat special foods to lose weight. I am much prouder of myself for eating the fresh *real* foods in the Salt Solution program."

Beth was very surprised to learn that when she fed her body properly, she wasn't hungry and didn't suffer her normal midafternoon energy slump. "It shocked me that when I followed the meals and timing, I wasn't hungry!" She also noticed that she no longer craved salt. "I feel so much better eating the meals outlined for me!" Beth loves the fact that her clothes are fitting better, but she also appreciates that the Salt Solution is a change she can make for life. "I am most pleased with the fact that I am losing weight in a way that makes me feel like I could continue this plan until I reach my goal."

Besides improving her weight (Beth lost 13 pounds in 6 weeks!), the Salt Solution improved Beth's life in other ways. "I feel like my ability to taste and appreciate the flavor of foods was improved." And she's started exercising regularly again, walking with a friend for an hour every morning.

SALT SOLUTION MAKEOVER

Beth's "**Before**" Diet

- **BREAKFAST:** Large serving of cereal with 2% milk, coffee with half-and-half
- **LUNCH:** Deli sandwich with cheese and mayonnaise, small handful of pretzels
- **SNACK:** Granola bar, coffee with half-and-half
- **DINNER:** Bratwurst, ravioli with tomato sauce, salad with ranch dressing
- **SNACK:** Chocolate pudding

"**Before**" Nutrition

- **Calories:** 2,559
- **Sodium:** 6,962 mg
- **Saturated Fat:** 43 g
- **Fiber:** 15 g

Beth's "**After**" Diet

- **BREAKFAST:** Spinach Scramble
- **LUNCH:** White Bean Hummus
- **SNACK:** Berry-Mango Smoothie
- **DINNER:** Mini Pizza with spinach salad and an apple
- **SNACK:** $\frac{1}{2}$ cup Greek yogurt frozen with lemon juice and Splenda

"**After**" Nutrition

- **Calories:** 1,315
- **Sodium:** 841 mg
- **Saturated Fat:** 10 g
- **Fiber:** 18 g

Salt Solution Improvements: Before the Salt Solution, Beth relied on processed deli meats, sausages, and prepared salad dressings and tomato sauces for meals—and her sodium intake was way too high as a consequence. After 6 weeks on the Salt Solution program, Beth drastically reduced her caloric intake (2,559 to 1,315 calories) and her sodium intake (6,962 mg sodium to 841 mg sodium). Not only does she look and feel fantastic, but her blood pressure dropped from 130/94 mmHg to a very healthy 115/82 mmHg—a sure consequence of slashing her sodium intake.

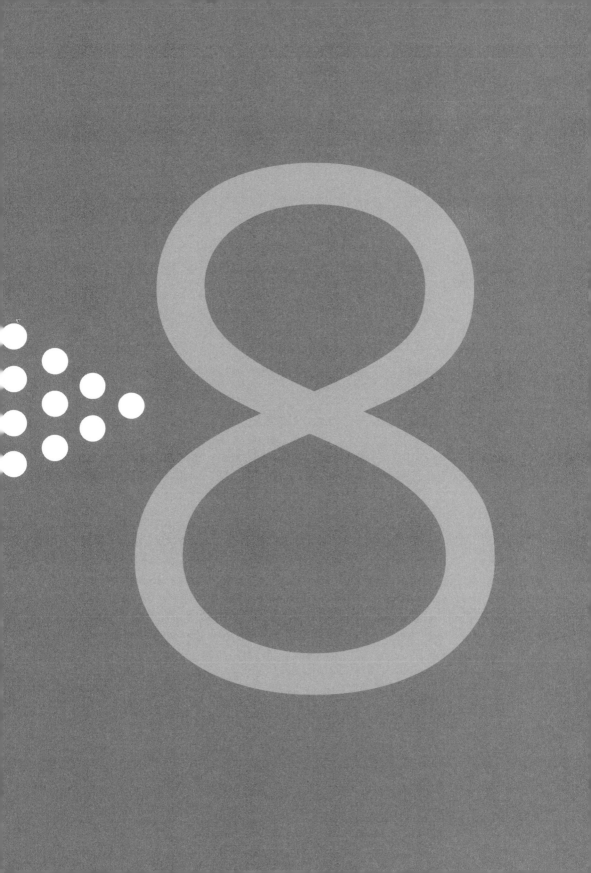

The Salt
SOLUTION
LIFESTYLE

Cleaning out the excess salt and calories from your diet (and your shopping cart) will improve your health and decrease your waistline, but there are other barriers that can stand in the way of your long-term weight-loss success.

You might have a busy schedule that leaves you grabbing fast food on the go, or an active social life that keeps you eating out more often than not. Maybe you have an emotional connection to food that drives you to devour a pint of ice cream or a jumbo bag of chips when you're feeling down or frazzled. Or perhaps you beat yourself up about your weight issues with negative self-talk. Although the problems we face differ for each of us, dealing with your diet-related issues is an important part of the healthful eating solution. In fact, we at *Prevention* know from years of research and observation that habits, mindset, and lifestyle choices can shape your success just as much as what you eat. That's why the Salt Solution is not just about cleaning out your diet, but also your mind, habits, and entire life.

The truth is, Americans live in a toxic food environment. We are surrounded by high-calorie, salty foods that are heavily promoted and hard to resist. Candy in the mall, doughnuts at the airport, hot dogs at the ball game, French fries on the boardwalk, pastries at the coffee shop, chips at service stations, dessert trays in restaurants, and fast food, well, everywhere! And, as in most cultures, food has tremendous social significance. People often eat so they can feel like they're part of the group, and for many the social pressure to eat is very powerful.

Whether it's cake at a birthday party, a burger at a summer barbecue, pie at Thanksgiving dinner, hors d'oeuvres at cocktail parties, or Aunt Mary insisting you have another piece of lasagna—some person, situation, or food will tempt you to stray from your Salt Solution eating plan. If you're weak in the willpower department, you'll be happy to hear that research shows that self-discipline is a type of mental muscle that grows stronger the more you use it. Put the following tactics into practice and you'll develop the type of resolve you need to eat, drink, and be merry, the Salt Solution way.

Dining Out Do's and Don'ts

WHETHER YOU'RE SHORT ON TIME or big on socializing, it's hard to avoid eating out. While controlling your sodium intake is easy when you prepare meals for yourself, things can get a little more complicated when someone else is doing the cooking. We already know that the majority of our salt intake comes from food not made at home, so you need to be on the lookout for meals that will cause your sodium intake to skyrocket. The bad news is that we can't always rely on our taste buds to indicate high-sodium meals. Salt is often hidden where we least expect it. Take this example: A Premium Caesar Salad with Grilled Chicken at McDonald's has more than double the sodium of a large order of fries (890 milligrams versus 350 milligrams).[1] A salad that's saltier than fries? It's true.

Fast-food chains are especially notorious for having high-sodium meals. Sandwiches and fast-food entrées can have up to 2,500 milligrams of sodium per serving—that's almost twice your daily allowance in just one Big Mac! And that's before you add the fries. Even a plain bagel (430 milligrams of sodium) and a caramel frappuccino (290 milligrams of sodium) can be salt-soaked. A recent study of meals from fast-food chains in New York has shown that they contain excessive amounts of salt, with more than half of all purchases exceeding the 1,500-milligram daily limit of sodium advised for most Americans.[2] Though a chain may not be able to prepare foods without salt for you since many of their foods are prepared in advance, you can still limit your sodium intake. Skip the cheese, go easy on condiments, avoid fried foods, and don't supersize anything, as this just means more calories, salt, and fat. To ensure a smaller portion, consider getting something off the children's menu. And, of course, limit fast food as much as possible.

Thankfully, though, you don't have to give up eating out in order to live the

Salt Solution lifestyle. There are many tips and tricks you can use to maximize your dining experience while minimizing your salt intake. The key is to plan and be proactive about what you're eating, using all the tools you've already acquired so far in this book. This may be easier to do at places where food is made to order instead of already prepared, but nothing is impossible!

So start by pushing that saltshaker away from you as soon as you're seated at the restaurant or fast-food joint. Now try these eating-out tips.

Don't Be Shy: Ask questions before ordering. Don't hold back. Ask how foods are prepared and don't hesitate to request that your meal be made without added salt, MSG, or salt-containing ingredients. Most restaurants are willing to accommodate requests. Feel free to bring your own low-sodium seasoning from home and sprinkle it on your meal if you want to spruce things up when your food arrives.

Top 10 Seriously Salty Foods at Restaurants

1. CHEESECAKE FACTORY'S FACTORY APPETIZER FAVORITES = 6,700 milligrams

2. CHILI'S JALAPENO SMOKEHOUSE BURGER WITH JALAPENO RANCH = 6,460 milligrams

3. APPLEBEE'S SIZZLING SKILLET SHRIMP FAJITAS = 6,060 milligrams

4. OUTBACK STEAKHOUSE BLOOMIN' ONION = 5,508 milligrams

5. RED LOBSTER ADMIRALS FEAST = 4,300 milligrams

6. CALIFORNIA PIZZA KITCHEN JAMAICAN JERK PIZZA = 4,236 milligrams

7. IHOP COUNTRY CHICKEN FRIED STEAK & EGGS WITH SAUSAGE GRAVY = 4,050 milligrams

8. RUBY TUESDAY SHRIMP CARBONARA PASTA CLASSIC = 3,766 milligrams

9. QUIZNOS CLASSIC ITALIAN LARGE SUB = 3,420 milligrams

10. ROMANO'S MACARONI GRILL SPAGHETTI & MEATBALLS BOLOGNESE = 3,040 milligrams

Cut the Condiments: They may mix up the flavor, but condiments also tend to load on the salt. So limit condiments, such as mustard, ketchup, sauces, and pickles. Once your taste buds are reset, you may find that condiments you formerly enjoyed now taste too salty, and you can do without them entirely. Don't hesitate to ask for them on the side so you can control how much you eat. Get salad dressings, sauces, and gravies on the side as well.

Skip the Bread: As we've learned, many baked goods contain salt, and bread is no exception. Why add extra calories and salt to your meal, especially since bread often fills you up before the main course? The tortilla chips you get at Mexican restaurants are no better; these are usually fried in fattening oil and highly salted. If you really can't resist the bread, however, at least make sure you ask for unsalted butter.

Watch Out for Red Flags: As you already know, soups and salad dressings often contain a lot of salt,

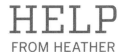

HELP
FROM HEATHER

Is your low-salt life a priority?

When you make something a priority, it becomes an important part of your life. Think back to one of your proudest accomplishments—whether it was starting a family, graduating from college, or landing your dream job. Remember the energy and commitment you employed in order to accomplish your goals? You rearranged your life in order to achieve success, and this same type of reprioritizing is essential in order for you to meet your weight-loss goals.

Do you prioritize the needs of others or your work obligations above your own health needs? What about your community duties or family responsibilities? Or do you think you're just too busy to make your own health a priority? The evidence is clear: Extra pounds combined with extra salt lead to a host of health issues, and most probably, a shortened life span. Don't wait until a health emergency forces you to make your weight loss and health a priority. A shift in priorities can be scary, but it is absolutely essential if you want to shake those extra pounds and cut the salt.

so try to avoid them. Casseroles, battered fried foods, rice pilaf, and dishes loaded with meat or cheese are also common sodium pitfalls. If an entrée comes with a sauce or gravy, that usually means a lot of sodium. Ask your server if these dishes can be made with less or no salt and to put sauces and gravy on the side. Better yet, steer clear of these options altogether. Smarter choices are meat, fish, and poultry that are grilled, broiled, steamed, or roasted without sauces or seasoning. You can get steamed veggies or a salad on the side.

Portion Control: If a menu contains only items with high salt, consider eating just half your meal and taking the rest for leftovers, or sharing dishes with a friend. Or ask if you can order a child's portion of a meal!

Plan Ahead: Doing a bit of research ahead of time can ensure that you'll already know your low-sodium options in advance and what questions you need to ask. This can help you make the best possible low-sodium choices, as well as avoid a last-minute meal decision that will lead to soaring sodium levels. Menu items change frequently, so go online to research the latest information. Many restaurants and fast-food chains have their menus available online, or you can ask for a nutrition fact sheet once you get there. Also, if you know

Words to Watch For

The description on the menu can tell you a lot about how a food is prepared. Don't forget those key words that tend to indicate "salty," such as *pickled, cured, smoked, soy sauce,* and *broth.* Stay away from these menu options. Words like *fried, battered, crispy, au gratin, scalloped,* and *creamed* usually mean big-time calories, plus trans or artery-clogging saturated fat. Instead, look for healthy key words like *grilled, baked, broiled,* or *dry roasted.*

ahead of time that you will be eating out later, you can go extra light on the sodium throughout the day so you can cheat a little more at night.

Mind over Matter

P EOPLE EAT FOR A LOT OF REASONS besides actual hunger—stress, boredom, sadness, and routine, just to name a few—and this is a surefire way to derail your diet. For many, the problem is in mindless eating. This is the type of eating you do automatically, without even noticing. According to a Cornell University study, when moviegoers were served popcorn in large buckets, they mindlessly munched 45 percent more than those given the same popcorn in medium-size containers.[3] Snacking on pretzels while watching TV, nibbling while you prepare food, grabbing a handful of candies every time you pass the reception desk—all this unconscious eating can add up to major calories and weight gain.

For others, the issue is emotional eating. When you're upset or lonely, do you reach for chocolate or cookies? If you've had a bad day, do you feel you've earned a big cheeseburger? For emotional eaters, food is more than just fuel—it's also a friend, a distraction, and a comfort. And when you're eating to squash your feelings or soothe your soul, it's all too easy to lose track of your intake and overeat.

Scientists, as we mentioned earlier, have discovered that some salty, fatty, and sugary foods (the type of fare that tends to accompany emotional and mindless eating, like the buttery, salty popcorn mentioned above) have an addictive quality that makes it hard to stop munching once you start. This makes unconscious eating a weight-loss double whammy! Being aware of *when* you eat, *why* you eat, and *what* you eat will not only help you control your mindless munching and emotional eating, but will also make it easier for you to make the best food choices possible. Here's how.

Get a Handle on Your Hunger

Ask yourself this: Can you tell the difference between physical hunger (hunger of the body) and phony hunger (hunger in the mind)? Being able to do so is an important first step in becoming a conscious eater. But it can be tricky. Here are some characteristics of each to help you distinguish between the two.

SIGNS OF PHYSICAL HUNGER (HUNGER OF THE BODY)

Comes on gradually

Accompanies a growling stomach

Open to food options

Stop eating when full

Can wait to be fed

Not associated with guilt

SIGNS OF PHONY HUNGER (HUNGER IN THE MIND)

Comes on suddenly

Accompanies a gnawing feeling of urgency

Craving for specific foods (chips, cookies, or whatever)

Eat past fullness

Must be fed immediately

Leaves guilt in its wake

Once you start paying attention to your hunger, you'll have an easier time distinguishing hunger in the mind from hunger of the body. If it's been a while since you've eaten because of actual physical hunger, use the hunger scale on the next page to help you out.

The Hunger Scale

0—Famished/Starving

1—Very Hungry

2—Slightly Hungry

3—Satisfied

4—Very Full

5—Stuffed!

Using this scale, notice when you're eating because of hunger (good) or as a result of boredom, emotional reasons, or simply because there is food available (not so good).

Sometimes just noticing your habitual responses can help break your automatic actions and reactions. Ultimately, you should start to eat at level 1 or 2, and stop eating when you reach level 3. If you begin at level 0, you're so hungry you're prone to overeat. If you go into a meal at 3 or above, you're likely eating out of boredom, stress, or some other emotional reason.

Write It Down!

A journal is a great tool to help you get a handle on your emotional eating and your sodium intake. In fact, in a recent study at the University of Kentucky and the University of North Carolina at Chapel Hill, scientists found that dieters who kept a journal tended to be more successful at weight loss than those who did not.[4] Tracking what you eat will help you discover your eating triggers and your sodium and calorie downfalls. *The Salt Solution Journal*, which you can buy at prevention.com/shop, has slots not only for your food and sodium intake, but also for when you ate, where you ate, and your hunger and emotional levels at the time. You might discover that your overeating occurs at night while you're surfing the Internet, or that you tend to reach for salty snacks most when "stressed about work" is jotted down in the emotions slot.

The more you use the food journal and the more accurately you record your intake, the more your journal will work for you! On page 347, you'll find instructions and general guidelines for filling out a food journal. You can copy the sample pages we've provided to use in the future or look for *The Salt Solution Journal* we've created for you at www.prevention.com/shop (or call 800-848-4735).

Focus on the Food

Mindless and emotional eaters have a tendency to zone out and lose track of their food consumption. They can eat an entire bag of chips and then feel the need to eat more simply because the food never registers with their senses. However, once you get your taste buds back into shape and learn to focus on your food, you'll find that meals are a whole lot more gratifying and weight loss is a whole lot easier. More good news: Although making a behavior change can be challenging, with some practice you can shift your focus and combat weight gain.

Follow a Schedule: Set aside designated meal times, and don't allow yourself to snack at any other times. Lucky for you we've done the work for you! The Salt Solution plan is designed with five minimeals each day, eaten with no more than 4 or 5 hours between meals, so you can lock yourself into eating delicious foods in the right quantity and at the right time.

Limit Distractions: Turn off the TV, put down your newspaper, shut off your computer, and just eat. Concentrate on the food's texture and flavor and truly enjoy the experience. After you reset your taste buds during the 2-Week

Cleanse, you'll be better able to savor the subtle flavors of your food—but only if you pay attention! Eat without distractions as often as possible, and when you feel ready, test your new skill in a restaurant. When you eat out, it's easy to get swept away in a conversation or the bustling atmosphere and to clean your plate without even noticing. But with a little patience, you can learn how to be a conscious eater no matter what the setting. Mastering this skill will take practice, but eventually it will click into place, much like riding a bike or driving a car, and you will be able to eat mindfully no matter what distractions surround you.

Eat Slowly: A recent study evaluated the eating habits of more than 3,000 people over 3 years. The conclusion? Those who ate at a fast rate were more likely to be overweight. Another study showed that women who ate their pasta lunch at a very fast rate (in just 9 minutes) ate 70 calories more than those who took their time (about half an hour). To help you slow down, put your fork down after each bite and don't pick it up again until you have swallowed. Try chewing each bite at least four or five times before swallowing and drinking water between bites. Doing so will help you eat less and, eventually, weigh less.

Attitude Adjustment

LOSING WEIGHT AND KEEPING IT OFF for good is about more than just shaking the salt, eating less, and exercising more. It's also about finding the right attitude. When you start a new diet plan and you slip up, how do you handle this roadblock? Do you brush it off and get back on track immediately? Or do you declare yourself a failure and break out the Cheetos? Or perhaps you have a small voice inside your head telling you your efforts to be healthy and lose weight are a waste of time—a voice that says things like:

"You can never lose weight. It's hopeless."

"I should just give up and eat that doughnut since I'll never lose weight."

"I always fail at this. Being fat must be in my genes."

A poor attitude can be just as damaging to your health as a high-salt, unhealthy diet. Spend a few days consciously listening to your inner voice and keeping a running tab of the negative messages you send to yourself. When you start thinking negative thoughts, do something for yourself—take a walk, read a book, call a friend—and ignore the voice. Be your own best

HELP
FROM HEATHER

Are you skipping meals?

Going too many hours between meals sends your blood sugar plummeting. That results in an out-of-control appetite that can leave your intentions to eat well in the dust. Suddenly every temptation becomes irresistible. Eating more often, on the other hand, maintains your energy levels, keeps your metabolism revved up, stabilizes your blood sugar, and controls your hunger, making it much easier for you to say no to that doughnut, slice of pizza, fried cheese stick, or other diet disaster. The Salt Solution plan is designed for you to have a small meal every 4 to 5 hours. By following this schedule, you'll prevent a sugar low that will leave you vulnerable to overindulging.

Need more reasons not to skip meals? Research shows that people who skip breakfast and eat fewer times during the day tend to be heavier than people who eat a healthy breakfast and eat four or five times a day. Another study showed that skipping meals and eating one large meal at night produced dangerous metabolic changes—including elevated blood sugar levels—that could lead to diabetes over the long term. And breakfast truly may be the most important meal of the day: Skipping breakfast has been associated with decreased physical activity and fewer calories burned overall during the day.

cheerleader instead, and you'll find your motivation and your weight loss will increase.

Give Yourself a Break: While it would be great if every day went fabulously and you stuck exactly to the letter of your diet, the truth is, nobody's perfect. Like any major change in life, losing weight and improving your health come with challenges. There are going to be a few days when something unexpected comes up—like a last-minute business dinner at a restaurant with tons of high-calorie, high-sodium menu items or a traffic jam that leaves you stranded with only fast food and convenience store lunch options. When something like this happens, don't beat yourself up over every occasional diet deal breaker. Just mark that slipup as an isolated mistake and get back onto the Salt Solution plan. It's more important to stick with the plan over the long haul than to be absolutely perfect over a period of a few days. After all, this is a long-term change you're making to lose weight and improve your health!

Give Yourself a Gift: You're about to do something fantastic for your health and appearance—and you deserve a reward! A nonfood indulgence will help you stay focused and motivated, and it's a great way to celebrate what you've accomplished. Small nonfood rewards, like a new bestseller, a CD of your favorite band, or an herb cooking class (to learn how to liven your food without salt), can help you celebrate steps like the end of the 2-Week Cleanse. When you complete the 4-Week Shake the Salt Meal Plan, consider a bigger reward, like a weekend vacation or a new outfit (to show off your new, leaner figure). The anticipated reward is sure to motivate you to reach the next milestone and stay positive.

Salt Solution Success Story

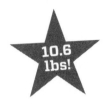

10.6 lbs!

Alice Mudge

Age: 60

Pounds Lost: 10.6

Inches Lost: 4¾ overall

A 60-YEAR-OLD ADMINISTRATIVE ASSISTANT, Alice had struggled with her weight for many years and had tried to drop the pounds many times before. But she was never able to stick to any of the diet programs for long. After she was diagnosed with diabetes in 2003, Alice knew she had to get her weight and eating patterns under control, but she continued to struggle. "I grew up in a family with five siblings, and we were never allowed to leave the table until our plates were clean. We had dessert every night—homemade pies, cinnamon rolls, and my grandmother's raised, deep-fried donuts." Naturally, Alice found it hard to break this ingrained pattern of eating and make lasting changes—until the Salt Solution.

"Now I'm much more aware of what I'm eating, portion size, and making better selections when I go out to eat." Alice plans her meals in advance and has discovered that she can follow the principles of the Salt Solution even when going on vacation or going out to eat with friends. She focuses on filling most of her plate with vegetables and fruit and watching portion sizes. "Now, I ask for a simple grilled chicken breast at restaurants. And I know to get melon slices instead of fries with my meal." Alice was most surprised at how satisfied she feels after eating the Salt Solution meals and how much she enjoys the flavor of food without adding salt.

After 6 weeks of the Salt Solution, Alice has found another benefit to the plan besides her 10.6-pound weight loss—blood sugar control. "I was amazed at how my blood sugar levels dropped while on the Salt Solution!"

SALT SOLUTION MAKEOVER

Alice's "**Before**" Diet

- **BREAKFAST:** Cheerios, ½ banana, ½ cup 2% milk
- **LUNCH:** Grilled cheese with tomato slices, potato chips, iced tea
- **DINNER:** Red Robin Whiskey River BBQ Chicken Burger with fries (½ portion—would share with a friend), iced tea

Alice's "**After**" Diet

- **BREAKFAST:** Berry Nut Topped Oatmeal
- **LUNCH:** Cranberries-on-a-Banana
- **DINNER:** 3-oz grilled steak, steamed broccoli, mango slices
- **SNACK:** Banana-Spinach Smoothie

"**Before**" Nutrition

- **Calories:** 2,005
- **Sodium:** 2,933 mg
- **Saturated Fat:** 30 g
- **Fiber:** 15 g

"**After**" Nutrition

- **Calories:** 1,464
- **Sodium:** 565
- **Saturated Fat:** 8 g
- **Fiber:** 14 g

Salt Solution Improvements: While Alice's caloric intake before starting the Salt Solution wasn't incredibly high, she was consuming too much sodium. After the Salt Solution, her sodium intake dropped sharply, from 2,933 mg to 565 mg. What Alice learned on the Salt Solution helped her lose almost 11 pounds in 6 weeks—and she's still going strong!

The Salt
SOLUTION
Weight-Loss
WORKOUT

Even though the Salt Solution eating plan is the fastest way to transform your body into the shape you've been hoping for, adding a little exercise into the equation can speed up the results—so you lose weight and look (and feel) better even faster. In addition, starting an exercise program could give you a little extra protection against high blood pressure, heart disease, diabetes, and all the other conditions associated with a high-sodium diet.

If the prospect of having to exercise scares you—because you have never exercised before, don't have enough time in your busy day, can't afford to make much of an investment in exercise equipment, or are simply nervous that what we're about to suggest may be too intense or overwhelming—don't worry.

We've created the ultimate way to burn off a few extra pounds—and boost your overall health simultaneously—that works for anyone, regardless of your schedule, fitness level, or lack of access to exercise equipment. Thanks to fitness expert Myatt Murphy, author of *The Body You Want in the Time You Have*, *The Men's Health Gym Bible*, and *Ultimate Dumbbell Guide*, we devised a companion workout that works not just with the Salt Solution eating plan but fits easily into any busy lifestyle. It's a workout plan that works with you, letting you decide how hard, or even how long, you want to exercise, so you're more likely to stick with the program and less likely to quit.

Why It Works

TO MAKE SURE YOU CAN STAY FOCUSED on this exercise program, we've designed it to incorporate a combination of several important fitness factors that make working out fun, easier, manageable, and more effective. This plan is:

Simple: There are virtually thousands of exercises you can use to get in shape, but certain exercises are more efficient at burning calories—and working more muscles at the same time—than others. To target as many muscles as possible within the shortest period of time, we've selected a series of multijoint, compound exercises and core-challenging poses that systemically work all your muscles from head to toe using just seven simple moves.

Adjustable: Unlike most workout programs that are designed to be a one-size-fits-all plan, this workout adapts to your fitness level. As you begin the plan, depending on your current physical abilities, you can either stick with it as prescribed, make it easier, or make it more challenging. That way, as you become more fit—or feel you may be pushing yourself too hard—you can instantly make adjustments to the program so you can continue to see results.

Low-Cost: All you need to perform this routine are a few exercise tools you probably already have in your closet: a pair of good walking shoes and 2 pairs of dumbbells of different weights (or a pair of adjustable dumbbells that allow you to reduce or add weight by stripping off or adding weight plates). If you find you want to raise the intensity of this workout at any time, there are a few additional pieces of fitness equipment you may need—such as a stability ball or exercise bench, for example—but to do the workout and get fast results, dumbbells are all you need.

Time-Saving: When it comes to strength training, most people work their muscles longer and harder than they really need to. Even though that might sound like the right formula for achieving faster results, it can easily leave you more sore and less interested in exercising—and can also increase your risk of injury. By mixing in a bit of science, we've developed a workout plan that keeps your heart and muscles constantly guessing, so they never get used to the routine. This strategy forces them to adapt faster, helping you get more muscle-building and fat-burning benefits in far less time than usual.

Together, these four factors do much more than simply spell S.A.L.T., they actually help make it easier to build muscle faster and stay motivated so you effortlessly stick with the program. The immediate results you'll see and feel from this workout will keep you from quitting, so you shed even more pounds and reach your target weight a lot sooner than you would if you followed the diet portion alone.

The Salt Solution Weight-Loss Workout Basics

THE WORKOUT YOU'LL BE FOLLOWING is actually a combination of two separate programs: a unique walking routine designed to burn fat fast and a strength-training routine tailored to boost your metabolism by raising your body's level of fat-burning lean muscle tissue.

To burn calories and blast body fat, you'll walk 6 days out of each week—with each day at a different tempo and length of time. To develop lean muscle, build core strength, and elevate your metabolism, you'll also be doing a strength-training regime 2 or 3 days per week—with each day designed with a different number of times you repeat each exercise as well as the amount of time you'll be resting between exercises.

Change Is Good

There's a reason each workout you do will be different each day. By constantly changing the way you walk/strength-train each day, you'll be less prone to boredom because each day will feel different, not only to you, but to your body as well. That difference also helps you build more lean muscle tissue and burn more calories, since your body will continuously have to adapt to each new workout as you change it around from day to day and week to week.

That's why you'll notice a gradual increase in how long and how hard you'll walk (or how many times you'll need to repeat certain exercises) week after week. As you lose more weight and feel healthier each and every week, your body will be ready for the next fitness milestone. Each new workout you'll be doing will account for those gains so your body is constantly challenged—and so the results keep coming.

Make It Work for You

The Salt Solution Weight-Loss Workout is highly effective if you follow both routines as prescribed in the overall program, but that doesn't mean you have to do exactly that.

The truth is, your fitness level may be much different from that of other dieters following this program, which is why tailoring a one-size-fits-all workout regime that addresses the fitness abilities of every possible type of dieter isn't easy. That's why this program works with you, letting you tweak it as you go to make it either less difficult if you're not quite in shape or more intense if you're already fit.

Every strength-training exercise in the program gives you the option of performing the move as described or making the exercise either easier or harder by letting you tweak it slightly. If any exercise is too difficult for you to do, just try the Make It Easier option instead. If any exercise is way too easy, then you can opt to do the Make It Harder option in its place. For even more flexibility, there are still more ways you can customize the workout even further to match your fitness level (see "Adjusting the Program for Your Fitness Level" on page 255).

If, for some reason, you simply don't have enough time to do both the walking and strength-training portions of the Salt Solution Weight-Loss Workout, then we recommend doing the walking portion only. If you prefer to do the strength-training portion only instead, that's fine, too. You'll lose less weight but gain more lean muscle (which will help your body burn more calories 24/7, even when you're at rest). However, keep in mind that doing both portions of the workout will yield the most results even faster than choosing one over the other.

The Best Order to Follow

If you're wondering if you should do the strength-training portion before or after the walking portion—or if you should wait a few hours between both workouts—that is entirely up to you. For best results (and only if time allows), here are the smartest options (in order of most effective).

1. Do the strength-training portion first, then wait a few hours before performing the walking portion. You'll elevate your metabolism twice instead of once that day, which can help burn a few extra calories each day.

2. If you would like to do both portions back-to-back to save time, start with the strength-training portion. That way, your muscles will be strong and fresh to handle the coordination needed to perform each exercise. Afterward, jump right into the walking portion.

Finally, before starting either routine in the Salt Solution Weight-Loss Workout, check with your doctor and follow his or her recommendations, especially if you have knee or joint problems, heart disease, foot problems, or other health concerns.

That said . . . let's get started!

The Salt Solution Walking Program

TO GET THE BEST RESULTS from each walking workout, you'll need to push yourself as much as required each day. That's not always easy to do—especially for a beginner—which is why the best way to gauge exactly how hard you're exercising is to use the Rate of Perceived Exertion (RPE) scale to be sure.

How to Do It: As you exercise, rate how hard you're exercising on a scale of 1 to 10 (one being "as little as possible" and 10 being "as hard as possible") by judging how well you can carry on a conversation as you go. Here's how to tell what level of exertion you're at as you exercise.

The Tempos You Need to Know

RPE 1-2 (VERY EASY): a very slow pace that allows you to carry on a conversation with no effort

RPE 3-4 (EASY TO MODERATELY EASY): a very easy pace that lets you carry on a conversation comfortably with minimum effort

RPE 5-6 (MODERATE TO MODERATELY HARD): a brisk pace that lets you talk, but it would be impossible to sing

RPE 7-8 (DIFFICULT TO VERY DIFFICULT): a high-intensity pace that lets you blurt out short phrases, but anything beyond that is impossible

RPE 9-10 (MAX EFFORT): an extremely high-intensity pace that makes carrying on a conversation virtually impossible

If you still can't decide how hard you're pushing yourself, counting the number of steps you can walk in exactly 1 minute may help. In a recent study performed at San Diego State University, researchers asked both male and female subjects to walk on a treadmill at various speeds, then monitored their oxygen uptake, step count, and heart rate. They found that when subjects reached what they determined to be a "moderate exercise level," men were walking at a rate of 92 to 102 steps per minute, while women ranged between 91 and 115 steps per minute.[1]

Although it may differ depending on your weight (and if you're walking on an incline, as opposed to a flat surface), the study results mean you're most likely reaching a 5 to 6 on the RPE scale if you're walking at a pace that falls between those numbers. Walking fewer steps per minute probably means you're exercising at a pace that's lower than a 5 to 6 on the RPE scale; walking more steps per minute probably means you're exercising at a pace that's higher than a 5 to 6 on the RPE scale.

The Walking Routines

THERE ARE FOUR UNIQUE STYLES OF WALKING that you'll be utilizing in the walking portion of the Salt Solution Weight-Loss Workout. They are as follows: Interval Walks, Steady-State Walks, Power Walks, and Recuperative Walks.

Why four?

Most walking routines stick with the same formula when it comes to time and intensity. As we mentioned earlier in this chapter, eventually, as your body gets used to the program, it will begin to learn how to do the routine in a more efficient manner that will cause you to use less energy and burn far less fat and fewer calories.

Using these four walking routines allows you to exercise at different intensities, which elevates your metabolism and burns stored fat in different ways. By combining all four into the same 6-week routine, you'll benefit by preventing your body from ever getting used to the demands you're placing on it, so it stays in a state of constant adaptation. That's why this regime targets more stored fat than the typical walking plan you may have tried with other diet programs in the past.

Here's how you'll perform each type of walking routine.

1. Interval Walks

After a 3- to 5-minute low-intensity warmup, you'll begin your first interval set by walking briskly for 3 minutes at a pace that's around 5 to 6 on the Rate of Perceived Exertion (RPE) scale.

Next, you'll speed up to a pace that's about a 7 to 8 on the RPE scale and walk for 1 minute. You'll repeat this pattern—3 minutes moderate intensity/ 1 minute high intensity—for the length of the workout (as prescribed). Afterward, you'll finish with a 3- to 5-minute cooldown walk.

2. Steady-State Walks

After a 3- to 5-minute low-intensity warmup, you'll walk at a tempo that's about a 5 on the RPE scale. You'll walk at this pace for the length of the workout (as prescribed), then finish with a 3- to 5-minute cooldown walk.

3. Power Walks

After a 3- to 5-minute low-intensity warmup, you'll begin walking at a pace that's roughly a 6 to 7 on the RPE scale. You'll walk at this pace for the length of the workout (as prescribed), then finish with a 3- to 5-minute cooldown walk.

4. Recuperative Walks

After a 3- to 5-minute, low-intensity warmup, you'll pick a comfortable moderate pace that you can easily walk for the prescribed amount of time. If you're tired from the week, stick with a tempo that's around a 4 on the RPE scale; if you have the energy, up the tempo to a 5 instead. You'll walk at this pace for the length of the workout (as prescribed), then finish with a 3- to 5-minute cooldown walk.

Note: This type of walking may seem similar to the Steady-State Walk at first, but these end-of-the-week walks are longer in length for several reasons.

First, because you'll be doing strength training 2 or 3 days during the week, you'll have less time then to devote to walking. But at the end of the week, you'll be given a nice 72- to 96-hour break from strength training, and this longer walk lets you take advantage of that extra free time to burn some additional calories.

Second, doing a nice longer-length walk will help you build up your endurance, which will make exercising a little bit easier to do each week.

Last, performing a low-intensity, long-duration aerobic activity will help your muscles flush out any remaining lactic acid (a waste product that collects in your muscles after weight lifting and causes a burning sensation) left over from the week's worth of strength training. This will help you recuperate a lot faster over the weekends, and you'll come back to each new week of workouts much more energized and less sore.

Beat the Heat to Melt More Pounds!

Exercising outdoors may feel refreshing, but not when it's too hot outside. Taking the right steps before and during your walking workouts will help you stay cool while firing up your metabolism. Just remember these five important rules before walking when it's hot outside.

1. CHOOSE THE RIGHT GEAR.

Tight-fitting clothes (especially those made from cotton) trap heat and moisture, and darker outfits absorb more sunlight and heat. Instead, wear lighter, looser-fitting clothing made from materials through which air can flow and that also draw moisture away from your body. (Some great materials to look for include Smartwool, Coolmax, and spun polyester.)

2. APPLY SUNSCREEN—EVEN IF IT'S CLOUDY.

Sunburn dehydrates your skin, which prevents your pores from working as effectively as they should. The more impaired they are, the less sweat you'll release and the hotter and more uncomfortable you'll feel as you walk. To protect yourself, always apply a sunscreen that's at least SPF 30 or higher and preferably one that's oil based rather than water based. (As you sweat, the oil-based sunscreen won't come off as easily, so you'll stay protected.)

3. WATCH THE CLOCK.

If possible, skip walking from 10 a.m. to 2 p.m. That's when the sun is at its highest, as are the ozone and UV ray levels. If you can, save your walks for either earlier in the morning, late afternoon, or early evening when the sun and its negative effects aren't at their peaks.

4. DIAL DOWN THE PACE.

Instead of exercising at your normal pace, try exercising at around 65 to 70 percent of your typical intensity or shorten your workout time by about one-third.

5. DRINK MORE THAN USUAL.

Before you exercise, drink at least 16 ounces of water, then drink at least 4 ounces of water every 15 minutes as you work out. Keeping yourself hydrated will help your body sweat more efficiently, which will help you feel cooler. After your workout, replace the sweat you've lost by drinking another 12 to 16 ounces of water.

Week 1

DAY ▷ INTERVAL WALK

1

Total Workout Time	The Routine	Intensity
35 minutes (25 minutes + 6 to 10 minutes for warmup and cooldown)	• 3- to 5-minute warmup	3–4
	• 3 minutes (brisk pace)	5–6
	• 1 minute (fast pace)	7–8
	• Continue to do 3-minute brisk/1-minute fast intervals 5 more times (for a total of 6 intervals)	5–6
	• 1 minute (brisk pace)	3–4
	• 3- to 5-minute cooldown	

DAY ▷ STEADY-STATE WALK

2

Total Workout Time	The Routine	Intensity
40 minutes (30 minutes + 6 to 10 minutes for warmup and cooldown)	• 3- to 5-minute warmup	3–4
	• 30 minutes (moderate pace)	5
	• 3- to 5-minute cooldown	3–4

DAY ▷ INTERVAL WALK

3

Total Workout Time	The Routine	Intensity
35 minutes (25 minutes + 6 to 10 minutes for warmup and cooldown)	• 3- to 5-minute warmup	3–4
	• 3 minutes (brisk pace)	5–6
	• 1 minute (fast pace)	7–8
	• Continue to do 3-minute brisk/1-minute fast intervals 5 more times (for a total of 6 intervals)	5–6
	• 1 minute (brisk pace)	3–4
	• 3- to 5-minute cooldown	

DAY ▷ POWER WALK

4

Total Workout Time	The Routine	Intensity
30 minutes (20 minutes + 6 to 10 minutes for warmup and cooldown)	• 3- to 5-minute warmup • 20 minutes (brisk/fast pace) • 3- to 5-minute cooldown	3–4 6–7 3–4

DAY ▷ INTERVAL WALK

5

Total Workout Time	The Routine	Intensity
35 minutes (25 minutes + 6 to 10 minutes for warmup and cooldown)	• 3- to 5-minute warmup • 3 minutes (brisk pace) • 1 minute (fast pace) • Continue to do 3-minute brisk/1-minute fast intervals 5 more times (for a total of 6 intervals) • 1 minute (brisk pace) • 3- to 5-minute cooldown	3–4 5–6 7–8 5–6 3–4

DAY ▷ RECUPERATIVE WALK

6

Total Workout Time	The Routine	Intensity
50 minutes (40 minutes + 6 to 10 minutes for warmup and cooldown)	• 3- to 5-minute warmup • 40 minutes (easy pace) • 3- to 5-minute cooldown	3–4 4 3–4

DAY ▷ REST

7

Week 2

▷ **INTERVAL WALK**

1

Total Workout Time	The Routine	Intensity
35 minutes (25 minutes + 6 to 10 minutes for warmup and cooldown)	• 3- to 5-minute warmup	3–4
	• 3 minutes (brisk pace)	5–6
	• 1 minute (fast pace)	7–8
	• Continue to do 3-minute brisk/1-minute fast intervals 5 more times (for a total of 6 intervals)	5–6
	• 1 minute (brisk pace)	3–4
	• 3- to 5-minute cooldown	

DAY ▷ **STEADY-STATE WALK**

2

Total Workout Time	The Routine	Intensity
40 minutes (30 minutes + 6 to 10 minutes for warmup and cooldown)	• 3- to 5-minute warmup	3–4
	• 30 minutes (moderate pace)	5
	• 3- to 5-minute cooldown	3–4

DAY ▷ **INTERVAL WALK**

3

Total Workout Time	The Routine	Intensity
35 minutes (25 minutes + 6 to 10 minutes for warmup and cooldown)	• 3- to 5-minute warmup	3–4
	• 3 minutes (brisk pace)	5–6
	• 1 minute (fast pace)	7–8
	• Continue to do 3-minute brisk/1-minute fast intervals 5 more times (for a total of 6 intervals)	5–6
	• 1 minute (brisk pace)	3–4
	• 3- to 5-minute cooldown	

DAY ⊳ **POWER WALK**

4

Total Workout Time	The Routine	Intensity
30 minutes (20 minutes + 6 to 10 minutes for warmup and cooldown)	• 3- to 5-minute warmup	3–4
	• 20 minutes (brisk/fast pace)	6–7
	• 3- to 5-minute cooldown	3–4

DAY ⊳ **INTERVAL WALK**

5

Total Workout Time	The Routine	Intensity
35 minutes (25 minutes + 6 to 10 minutes for warmup and cooldown)	• 3- to 5-minute warmup	3–4
	• 3 minutes (brisk pace)	5–6
	• 1 minute (fast pace)	7–8
	• Continue to do 3-minute brisk/1-minute fast intervals 5 more times (for a total of 6 intervals)	5–6
	• 1 minute (brisk pace)	3–4
	• 3- to 5-minute cooldown	

DAY ⊳ **RECUPERATIVE WALK**

6

Total Workout Time	The Routine	Intensity
1 hour (50 minutes + 6 to 10 minutes for warmup and cooldown)	• 3- to 5-minute warmup	3–4
	• 50 minutes (easy pace)	4
	• 3- to 5-minute cooldown	3–4

DAY ⊳ **REST**

7

Week 3

▷ **INTERVAL WALK**

1

Total Workout Time	The Routine	Intensity
40 minutes (30 minutes + 6 to 10 minutes for warmup and cooldown)	• 3- to 5-minute warmup	3–4
	• 3 minutes (brisk pace)	5–6
	• 1 minute (fast pace)	7–8
	• Continue to do 3-minute brisk/1-minute fast intervals 6 more times (for a total of 7 intervals)	5–6
	• 2 minutes (brisk pace)	3–4
	• 3- to 5-minute cooldown	

DAY ▷ **STEADY-STATE WALK**

2

Total Workout Time	The Routine	Intensity
55 minutes (45 minutes + 6 to 10 minutes for warmup and cooldown)	• 3- to 5-minute warmup	3–4
	• 45 minutes (moderate pace)	5
	• 3- to 5-minute cooldown	3–4

DAY ▷ **INTERVAL WALK**

3

Total Workout Time	The Routine	Intensity
40 minutes (30 minutes + 6 to 10 minutes for warmup and cooldown)	• 3- to 5-minute warmup	3–4
	• 3 minutes (brisk pace)	5–6
	• 1 minute (fast pace)	7–8
	• Continue to do 3-minute brisk/1-minute fast intervals 6 more times (for a total of 7 intervals)	5–6
	• 2 minutes (brisk pace)	3–4
	• 3- to 5-minute cooldown	

DAY 4 ▷ POWER WALK

Total Workout Time	The Routine	Intensity
40 minutes (30 minutes + 6 to 10 minutes for warmup and cooldown)	• 3- to 5-minute warmup • 30 minutes (brisk/fast pace) • 3- to 5-minute cooldown	3–4 6–7 3–4

DAY 5 ▷ INTERVAL WALK

Total Workout Time	The Routine	Intensity
40 minutes (30 minutes + 6 to 10 minutes for warmup and cooldown)	• 3- to 5-minute warmup • 3 minutes (brisk pace) • 1 minute (fast pace) • Continue to do 3-minute brisk/1-minute fast intervals 6 more times (for a total of 7 intervals) • 2 minutes (brisk pace) • 3- to 5-minute cooldown	3–4 5–6 7–8 5–6 3–4

DAY 6 ▷ RECUPERATIVE WALK

Total Workout Time	The Routine	Intensity
1 hour 10 minutes (1 hour + 6 to 10 minutes for warmup and cooldown)	• 3- to 5-minute warmup • 1 hour (easy pace) • 3- to 5-minute cooldown	3–4 4 3–4

DAY 7 ▷ REST

Week 4

INTERVAL WALK

1

Total Workout Time	The Routine	Intensity
40 minutes (30 minutes + 6 to 10 minutes for warmup and cooldown)	• 3- to 5-minute warmup	3–4
	• 3 minutes (brisk pace)	5–6
	• 1 minute (fast pace)	7–8
	• Continue to do 3-minute brisk/1-minute fast intervals 6 more times (for a total of 7 intervals)	5–6
	• 2 minutes (brisk pace)	3–4
	• 3- to 5-minute cooldown	

DAY ▷ **STEADY-STATE WALK**

2

Total Workout Time	The Routine	Intensity
55 minutes (45 minutes + 6 to 10 minutes for warmup and cooldown)	• 3- to 5-minute warmup	3–4
	• 45 minutes (moderate pace)	5
	• 3- to 5-minute cooldown	3–4

DAY ▷ **INTERVAL WALK**

3

Total Workout Time	The Routine	Intensity
40 minutes (30 minutes + 6 to 10 minutes for warmup and cooldown)	• 3- to 5-minute warmup	3–4
	• 3 minutes (brisk pace)	5–6
	• 1 minute (fast pace)	7–8
	• Continue to do 3-minute brisk/1-minute fast intervals 6 more times (for a total of 7 intervals)	5–6
	• 2 minutes (brisk pace)	3–4
	• 3- to 5-minute cooldown	

DAY ▷ POWER WALK

4

Total Workout Time	The Routine	Intensity
40 minutes (30 minutes + 6 to 10 minutes for warmup and cooldown)	• 3- to 5-minute warmup • 30 minutes (brisk/fast pace) • 3- to 5-minute cooldown	3–4 6–7 3–4

DAY ▷ INTERVAL WALK

5

Total Workout Time	The Routine	Intensity
40 minutes (30 minutes + 6 to 10 minutes for warmup and cooldown)	• 3- to 5-minute warmup • 3 minutes (brisk pace) • 1 minute (fast pace) • Continue to do 3-minute brisk/1-minute fast intervals 6 more times (for a total of 7 intervals) • 2 minutes (brisk pace) • 3- to 5-minute cooldown	3–4 5–6 7–8 5–6 3–4

DAY ▷ RECUPERATIVE WALK

6

Total Workout Time	The Routine	Intensity
1 hour 20 minutes (1 hour 10 minutes + 6 to 10 minutes for warmup and cooldown)	• 3- to 5-minute warmup • 1 hour 10 minutes (easy pace) • 3- to 5-minute cooldown	3–4 4 3–4

DAY ▷ REST

7

Week 5

INTERVAL WALK

1

Total Workout Time	The Routine	Intensity
45 minutes (35 minutes + 6 to 10 minutes for warmup and cooldown)	• 3- to 5-minute warmup	3–4
	• 3 minutes (brisk pace)	5–6
	• 1 minute (fast pace)	7–8
	• Continue to do 3-minute brisk/1-minute fast intervals 7 more times (for a total of 8 intervals)	5–6
	• 3 minutes (brisk pace)	3–4
	• 3- to 5-minute cooldown	

DAY ▷ **STEADY-STATE WALK**

2

Total Workout Time	The Routine	Intensity
1 hour 10 minutes (1 hour + 6 to 10 minutes for warmup and cooldown)	• 3- to 5-minute warmup	3–4
	• 1 hour (moderate pace)	5
	• 3- to 5-minute cooldown	3–4

DAY ▷ **INTERVAL WALK**

3

Total Workout Time	The Routine	Intensity
45 minutes (35 minutes + 6 to 10 minutes for warmup and cooldown)	• 3- to 5-minute warmup	3–4
	• 3 minutes (brisk pace)	5–6
	• 1 minute (fast pace)	7–8
	• Continue to do 3-minute brisk/1-minute fast intervals 7 more times (for a total of 8 intervals)	5–6
	• 3 minutes (brisk pace)	3–4
	• 3- to 5-minute cooldown	

DAY 4 ▶ POWER WALK

Total Workout Time	The Routine	Intensity
50 minutes (40 minutes + 6 to 10 minutes for warmup and cooldown)	• 3- to 5-minute warmup • 40 minutes (brisk/fast pace) • 3- to 5-minute cooldown	3–4 6–7 3–4

DAY 5 ▶ INTERVAL WALK

Total Workout Time	The Routine	Intensity
45 minutes (35 minutes + 6 to 10 minutes for warmup and cooldown)	• 3- to 5-minute warmup • 3 minutes (brisk pace) • 1 minute (fast pace) • Continue to do 3-minute brisk/1-minute fast intervals 7 more times (for a total of 8 intervals) • 3 minutes (brisk pace) • 3- to 5-minute cooldown	3–4 5–6 7–8 5–6 3–4

DAY 6 ▶ RECUPERATIVE WALK

Total Workout Time	The Routine	Intensity
1 hour 30 minutes (1 hour 20 minutes + 6 to 10 minutes for warmup and cooldown)	• 3- to 5-minute warmup • 1 hour 20 minutes (easy pace) • 3- to 5-minute cooldown	3–4 4 3–4

DAY 7 ▶ REST

Week 6

1

Total Workout Time	The Routine	Intensity
45 minutes (35 minutes + 6 to 10 minutes for warmup and cooldown)	• 3- to 5-minute warmup	3–4
	• 3 minutes (brisk pace)	5–6
	• 1 minute (fast pace)	7–8
	• Continue to do 3-minute brisk/1-minute fast intervals 7 more times (for a total of 8 intervals)	5–6
	• 3 minutes (brisk pace)	3–4
	• 3- to 5-minute cooldown	

DAY ▷ **STEADY-STATE WALK**

2

Total Workout Time	The Routine	Intensity
1 hour 10 minutes (1 hour + 6 to 10 minutes for warmup and cooldown)	• 3- to 5-minute warmup	3–4
	• 1 hour (moderate pace)	5
	• 3- to 5-minute cooldown	3–4

DAY ▷ **INTERVAL WALK**

3

Total Workout Time	The Routine	Intensity
45 minutes (35 minutes + 6 to 10 minutes for warmup and cooldown)	• 3- to 5-minute warmup	3–4
	• 3 minutes (brisk pace)	5–6
	• 1 minute (fast pace)	7–8
	• Continue to do 3-minute brisk/1-minute fast intervals 7 more times (for a total of 8 intervals)	5–6
	• 3 minutes (brisk pace)	3–4
	• 3- to 5-minute cooldown	

DAY ▷ **POWER WALK**

4

Total Workout Time	The Routine	Intensity
50 minutes (40 minutes + 6 to 10 minutes for warmup and cooldown)	• 3- to 5-minute warmup • 40 minutes (brisk/fast pace) • 3- to 5-minute cooldown	3–4 6–7 3–4

DAY ▷ **INTERVAL WALK**

5

Total Workout Time	The Routine	Intensity
45 minutes (35 minutes + 6 to 10 minutes for warmup and cooldown)	• 3- to 5-minute warmup • 3 minutes (brisk pace) • 1 minute (fast pace) • Continue to do 3-minute brisk/1-minute fast intervals 7 more times (for a total of 8 intervals) • 3 minutes (brisk pace) • 3- to 5-minute cooldown	3–4 5–6 7–8 5–6 3–4

DAY ▷ **RECUPERATIVE WALK**

6

Total Workout Time	The Routine	Intensity
1 hour 40 minutes (1 hour 30 minutes + 6 to 10 minutes for warmup and cooldown)	• 3- to 5-minute warmup • 1 hour 30 minutes (easy pace) • 3- to 5-minute cooldown	3–4 4 3–4

DAY ▷ **REST**

7

The Salt Solution Strength-Training Routine

N ADDITION TO WALKING, you'll also be performing a strength-training routine 2 or 3 days a week in order to develop lean muscle, build core strength, and elevate your metabolism.

The strength-training portion of the Salt Solution Weight-Loss Workout is a specifically crafted routine that combines just seven exercises designed to collectively work all your muscles from head to toe in the shortest amount of time. When it comes to training your body to be a fat-burning machine, it's the largest muscles in your body—especially your quadriceps, hamstrings, gluteal muscles, back, and chest—that should demand the most attention. Increasing your overall lean muscle mass raises your resting metabolic rate, that is, the amount of calories your body burns all day long. That's why targeting your larger muscles, not just specific ones you want to get in shape, plays a big part in helping you burn the greatest number of calories. This routine does just that, so you build more muscle—and burn more calories, even when you're at rest, at work, or even in bed fast asleep.

Strength-Training Basics

F YOU'VE NEVER USED DUMBBELLS BEFORE or it's been a while since you've performed any strength-training exercises, you'll need to know a few weight-lifting rules to start.

First, the word *rep* is short for repetition, which means performing an exercise once. A specific number of reps (8, 10, 12, or 15, for example) is called a set. So, for example, if you're asked to perform two sets of 15 reps of

Adjusting the Program
for Your Fitness Level

All the exercise routines within the Salt Solution Weight-Loss Workout are designed to deliver maximum results. However, if you're new to exercise or feel more comfortable easing into the program at your own pace, there are a few simple steps you can do to dial back the intensity so that it works within your own comfort zone.

WITH EVERY WALKING WORKOUT:

- Instead of doing the number of minutes suggested for each day, you can divide that number by half. (For example, if the program asks you to walk for 30 minutes, try walking for 15 minutes instead.) As the weeks progress and you gradually become more fit, you can begin adding a few extra minutes back into your workouts until you eventually feel comfortable exercising for the recommended time.

- If the length of any walking workout is too long for you to complete timewise because of your schedule, simply split the workout up into 2 segments.

(For example, if you can't walk for the recommended 40 minutes one day, try breaking your workout up into two 20-minute walks instead.)

WITH EVERY STRENGTH-TRAINING EXERCISE:

- As you follow all 6 weeks of the Salt Solution Weight-Loss Workout, you'll gradually begin to do more and more sets of the exercises. However, if the number of sets is too much for you—either because of time or intensity—then simply do 1 less set per exercise. (For example, if you're asked to do 2 sets of an exercise, try doing 1 set instead.)

- In between each exercise, the Salt Solution Weight-Loss Workout instructs you to rest for a certain number of seconds to allow your muscles to recover. However, if the pace of the workout feels too intense, try resting an additional 15 to 30 seconds between each set to catch your breath.

an exercise, that means you'll do that exercise 15 times (that's one set), then perform the exercise again 15 times (you'll be instructed how long to rest in between each set in each workout). A few other rules to keep in mind:

If you have never done any strength-training exercises, haven't exercised in more than 6 months, or have any pre-existing knee problems, start with the "Make It Easier" option. Otherwise, start with the original exercise. If that's too difficult, perform the "Make It Easier" option. If it's not hard enough, perform the "Make It Harder" option.

Before you start the program, always warm up your muscles first by walking at an easy pace (3 to 4 RPE) for 4 to 5 minutes.

Do each exercise in the exact numerical order listed in the program.

For each exercise, try to maintain a comfortable pace that allows you to raise the weight in 2 seconds and lower it in 2 seconds. Rushing through each exercise any faster will only increase your risk of injury.

Each day, you'll follow the instructions in the chart on how many sets/repetitions to do of each exercise (as well as how many seconds to rest in between

Sweat More to Age Less

Not only can the Salt Solution Weight-Loss Workout help you look thinner, but it could also help you age more slowly. A recent study performed at the University of California, San Francisco,[2] found that exercise helps to prevent telomeres—the tiny pieces of DNA that protect your chromosomes—from shortening and unraveling from stress. According to their findings, even brief vigorous exercise (as little as 42 minutes over a 3-day period) may reduce the effects of stress-induced cell aging.

each set). Do the required amount of sets for each exercise before moving onto the next exercise.

How Much Weight Should You Use?

For each exercise, you want to start with a moderate weight that lets you perform the required amount of repetitions. If you can do more reps than recommended, you need to increase the amount of weight you're lifting. If you can't do at least 8 reps, then the weight is too heavy. Choose a lighter weight or try the easier version of the exercise.

Note: Because some muscles are bigger than others, you'll need to use heavier dumbbells for exercises that target your chest, back, legs, and butt. For smaller muscles like your arms and shoulders, you'll probably want to choose lighter dumbbells.

Our recommendation for maximum results: A few days before you start the program, try giving each exercise a test run and do a sample set of each move. If you're a beginner, start by using 3- to 5-pound dumbbells, just to be safe. Advanced exercisers can start with 5- to 8-pound dumbbells. You should be able to gauge if the weight you're using is too light or too heavy, or if you need to change the exercise either by using the "Make It Easier" move or the "Make It Harder" move. That way, when you start the program, you'll be more likely to start off using the amount of weight and the variation of each exercise that works best for you.

Final safety note: If you think that using the heaviest weight you can handle will yield even more results, please don't take that risk. Choosing weights that are too heavy for you to handle will only increase your risk of injury, which could cause you to quit the program before it has a chance to work with the diet. Instead, be smart and pick a weight that follows the above recommendations.

THE 6-WEEK STRENGTH-TRAINING PLAN

WEEK	DAY 1	DAY 2	DAY 3	DAY 4	DAY 5	DAY 6	DAY 7
1	OFF	2 sets, 15 reps, 45–60 seconds rest	OFF	OFF	2 sets, 15 reps, 45–60 seconds rest	OFF	OFF
2	OFF	2 sets, 12 reps, 30–45 seconds rest	OFF	OFF	2 sets, 12 reps, 30–45 seconds rest	OFF	OFF
3	2 sets, 15 reps, 45–60 seconds rest	OFF	2 sets, 12 reps, 30–45 seconds rest	OFF	2 sets, 10 reps, 15–30 seconds rest	OFF	OFF
4	2 sets, 15 reps, 45–60 seconds rest	OFF	2 sets, 12 reps, 30–45 seconds rest	OFF	2 sets, 10 reps, 15–30 seconds rest	OFF	OFF
5	3 sets, 15 reps, 45–60 seconds rest	OFF	3 sets, 12 reps, 30–45 seconds rest	OFF	3 sets, 10 reps, 15–30 seconds rest	OFF	OFF
6	3 sets, 15 reps, 45–60 seconds rest	OFF	3 sets, 12 reps, 30–45 seconds rest	OFF	3 sets, 10 reps, 15–30 seconds rest	OFF	OFF

Four Bonus Benefits

The Salt Solution Weight-Loss Workout isn't just effective for shedding unwanted pounds and boosting your overall health. Here are four science-backed advantages to following the program that you'll see and feel now—and for years to come!

● **Sounder sleep:** According to a recent study[3] from the Institute of Exercise and Health Sciences at the University of Basel, subjects who believed they weren't exercising enough didn't sleep as well as subjects who perceived that they were fit. That means if using the Salt Solution Weight-Loss Workout makes you feel fitter, you'll sleep better.

● **Appetite reduction:** A study performed by the University of Colorado Denver discovered that regular exercise actually prevented weight gain after dieting by causing the body to burn fat first over carbohydrates.[4] This may help signal a feeling of fullness to the brain, which in turn could cause you to be less likely to overeat.

● **Lifted spirits:** Going outside when performing the walking portion of the Salt Solution Weight-Loss Workout has been shown to elevate your mood. A recent UK study[5] found that just 5 minutes of exercise in a park, on a nature trail, or in any other green space improved a person's mood and sense of well-being.

● **Trimmer tummy:** Looking to keep the belly fat you've lost from the Salt Solution Diet away for good? Exercise physiologists at the University of Alabama at Birmingham (UAB) Department of Human Studies[6] found that just 80 minutes a week of aerobic or resistance training not only helped prevent weight gain, but subjects regained zero percent of harmful visceral fat— the deadly fat that surrounds your organs—1 year after weight loss.

THE EXERCISES

1. Squat Sweep

(works the quadriceps, hamstrings, inner thighs, and glutes)

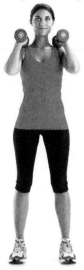

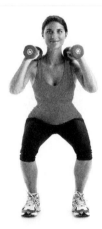

START POSITION: Stand with your feet shoulder-width apart holding a dumbbell in each hand. Curl the weights up until the ends rest on the front of your shoulders.

A. Keeping your back straight, slowly bend your hips and sit back until your thighs are almost parallel to the floor.

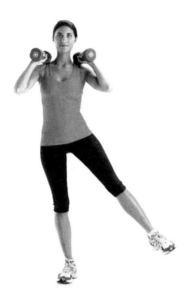

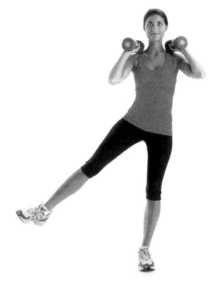

B. As you stand back up, lift your left leg straight out to your side as if you were going to step out. Shoot for raising your foot about 6 inches off the floor, but avoid raising your leg any higher than hip height. Pause for 1 second, then return your foot to the floor so you're back in the start position.

C. Repeat the exercise, this time lifting your right leg out to the side.

D. Alternate legs between every squat for the entire set.

MAKE IT EASIER: Perform the exercise without weights, or try squatting down about half the distance during each repetition.

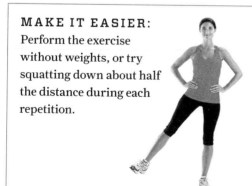

MAKE IT HARDER: Instead of taking 2 seconds to squat down and 2 seconds to stand back up (as recommended in the Strength-Training Basics on page 254), go twice as slow (4 seconds down/ 4 seconds up).

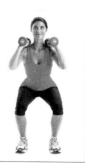

2. Double Chest Press + Fly

(works the chest, shoulders, and triceps)

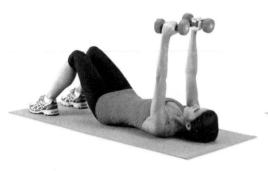

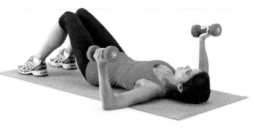

START POSITION: Lie face up on the floor (or a bench) holding a light dumbbell in each hand, knees bent, feet flat on the floor. Raise your arms straight above your chest, with your palms facing each other.

A. Bend your elbows out to your sides and slowly lower the weights until your upper arms touch the floor. (Your palms should stay facing each other as you go.)

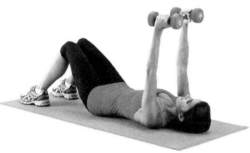

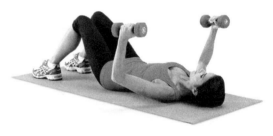

B. Press the weights back up into the start position, then repeat the move once more. This is the chest press.

C. Next, slowly sweep your arms out to your sides and down as far as you can. Reverse the motion by sweeping your arms back up in front of you (as if you're hugging someone) until they're back in the start position. This is the fly. Alternate between 2 presses and 1 fly for the recommended amount of repetitions.

MAKE IT EASIER: Once your upper arms touch the floor, rest for 1 second before pushing the weights back into the start position.

MAKE IT HARDER: Lie on a stability ball with your head, shoulders, and upper back supported by the ball; your knees should be bent and your feet flat on the floor. Your body should be one straight line from your head to your knees.

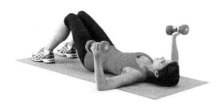

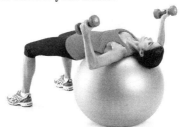

3. Lunge

(works the quadriceps, hamstrings, and glutes)

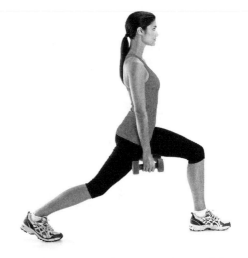

START POSITION: Stand straight with a dumbbell in each hand, your arms hanging straight down from your sides, and your palms facing in.

A. Take a big step forward with your left foot and lower your body until your left thigh is almost parallel to the floor. (Your right leg should be extended behind you with only the ball of your right foot on the floor.)

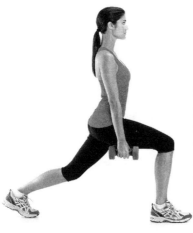

B. Reverse the motion by pressing yourself back into the start position, then repeat the exercise by stepping forward with your right foot. Alternate between stepping forward with your left and right feet throughout the set.

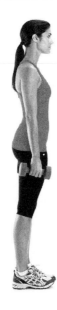

MAKE IT EASIER: Do the exercise without any weights (hands on hips), or try a reverse lunge instead. Stand with your feet together, then step back about 2 to 3 feet with your right foot. Bend your left knee and slowly lower yourself down. (Your left knee should stay directly over your ankle.) Stop right before your right knee touches the floor, then push off with your right foot to get back into the start position. Repeat the move with your left leg.

MAKE IT HARDER: Try turning the movement into a traveling lunge. Instead of stepping back into the start position, keep your front foot planted, then bring the leg that's behind you forward and raise your knee up in front of you. (You'll be balancing on just your front leg.) Plant your foot back down so your feet are even once more.

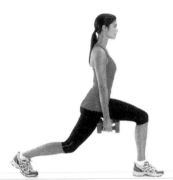

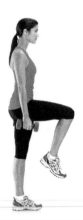

4. Unilateral Bent-Over Row

(works the latissimus dorsi, rhomboids, lower back, and core)

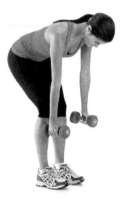 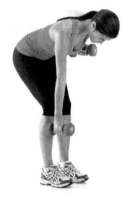

START POSITION: Stand with your feet shoulder-width apart, holding a light dumbbell in each hand with an overhand grip, knees slightly bent. Bend forward at your hips until your torso is almost parallel to the floor. Your arms should be hanging straight beneath you, palms facing each other.

A. Keeping your elbows close to your body, pull the weight in your left hand up to the side of your chest. (Your right arm will stay straight.)

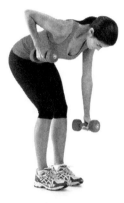

B. Lower the weight in your left hand back down as you simultaneously pull the weight in your right hand up to your side. Continue alternating back and forth for the entire set.

MAKE IT EASIER: Try doing the exercise one arm at a time. To support your lower back, place one hand on a sturdy chair, then bend forward until your torso is at a 45-degree angle to the floor. Do the required repetitions for one arm, then switch positions to work your other arm.

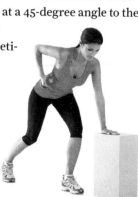

MAKE IT HARDER: Every 1 or 2 repetitions, pull both weights up along your sides, then push your heels into the floor and straighten back up into a standing position, keeping the weights locked into your sides as you go. Immediately reverse the motion, bend forward at the waist first, then lower the weights back down by straightening your arms.

5. Deadlift Curl Press

(works the trapezius, lower back, glutes, hamstrings, shoulders, triceps, and biceps)

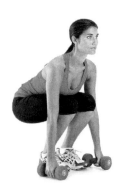

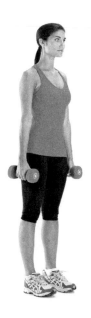

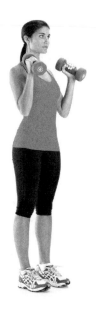

START POSITION: Stand with your feet spaced 6 to 8 inches apart with a dumbbell placed along the outside of each foot. Bend your knees and grab the dumbbells so that your palms face in toward each other. Before you begin the exercise, make sure that your back and shoulders are straight (not rounded) and your head is up.

A. Keeping your head and back straight, slowly stand up until your legs are straight, knees unlocked, keeping the dumbbells close to your body as you lift.

B. Without moving your upper arms, bend your elbows and curl the weights up to the front of your shoulders, palms facing each other.

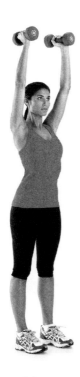

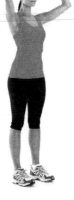

MAKE IT EASIER: Instead of starting the exercise with the weights on the floor, place them on a pair of sturdy boxes. This will prevent you from having to lower yourself down as far, which makes the move much simpler to perform.

MAKE IT HARDER: Try pausing a few times during the exercise. This will keep your muscles under a longer duration of tension so you utilize even more muscle fibers. During each repetition:

- Pause for 1 second during the deadlift portion (when your thighs are at a 45-degree angle as you rise up).
- Pause for 1 second during the curl portion (when your forearms are parallel to the floor).
- Pause for 1 second during the pressing portion (when your arms are bent at 90-degree angles).

C. Press the weights up over your head until your arms are straight, elbows unlocked, palms facing each other. Reverse the entire exercise until you're back in the start position.

6. Bicycle Crunch

(works the abdominal muscles)

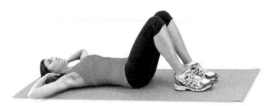

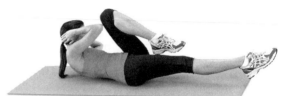

START POSITION: Lie face up on the floor with your knees bent and your feet flat on the floor. Lightly cup your hands over your ears, letting your elbows point out to the sides.

A. Draw your left knee toward your chest while simultaneously extending your right leg. Simultaneously curl your torso up and twist to the left, so that your right elbow and left knee touch (or at least come close to touching).

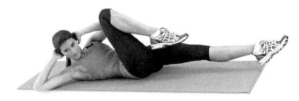

B. Repeat the exercise (this time pulling your right knee in as you curl and twist your torso to the right, touching your left elbow to your right knee). Alternate back and forth from side to side for the entire exercise, keeping your feet off the floor the entire time.

MAKE IT EASIER: Keep your knees bent and your feet on the floor, then raise only one knee at a time, leaving the opposite foot on the floor.

MAKE IT HARDER: Try pausing for 1 or 2 seconds each time your elbow meets your knee. Or better yet, pulse by doing 1 or 2 minireps (bringing your knee and elbow together, then apart by an inch or so, then back together again). Either way will keep your abs contracted for a longer period of time.

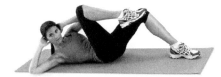
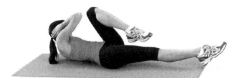

7. Plank

(works the core muscles)

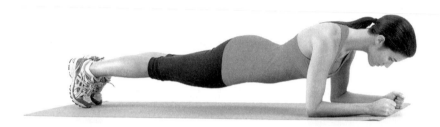

START POSITION: Get into a pushup position—legs extended behind you, feet shoulder-width apart, with your weight on your toes. Rest on your forearms so that your arms are at 90-degree angles.

Keeping your head and back straight, hold this position for the prescribed amount of time. (For Week 1, hold for 30 seconds; for each additional week, add between 5 and 10 seconds, depending on your strength level.)

MAKE IT EASIER: Bend your legs so that you're resting on one knee (your other leg stays extended) or both knees.

MAKE IT HARDER: Instead of staying in place, keep your arms and feet in place, then slowly twist and lower your left hip toward the floor. Repeat by twisting the opposite way and lowering your right hip. Alternate back and forth for the entire duration.

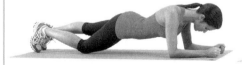

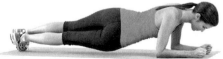

Use Your Brain to Help Burn Fat!

You can reap even more from this program by placing yourself in the right frame of mind. All it takes is understanding why some people succeed with most exercise programs—and why many people fail—to stay on course so you continuously lose weight and get lean even faster.

THOSE THAT SEE MORE RESULTS . . . listen to their bodies as they exercise.
THOSE THAT SEE FEWER RESULTS . . . ignore or push through the wrong types of pain. (Muscle soreness is normal, but if you feel stress in your joints or experience any form of pain, stop immediately, then reexamine how hard you're pushing yourself and/or if you're doing the move incorrectly.)

THOSE THAT SEE MORE RESULTS . . . know that body fat comes off differently from person to person.
THOSE THAT SEE FEWER RESULTS . . . think they can remove fat from certain areas. (Believing you can spot reduce fat can disappoint you, especially if you aren't losing weight exactly where you want to right away. Don't worry. Stick to the plan and you'll see it disappear from all of your trouble spots soon enough.)

THOSE THAT SEE MORE RESULTS . . . are willing to try something new (like this program).
THOSE THAT SEE FEWER RESULTS . . . stick with the same routine for months. (Even if you are currently using an exercise program, trying our plan will shake things up for your muscles. It's a trick that forces your body to adapt to something new, which causes it to burn even more calories.)

THOSE THAT SEE MORE RESULTS . . . always have a backup plan when life gets in the way of exercise.
THOSE THAT SEE FEWER RESULTS . . . skip exercising when they can't do exactly what they're told. (Even though we've laid out the perfect exercise plan to complement your diet program, don't be afraid to substitute doing something active that also burns calories if a busy day prevents you from either walking or strength-training.)

THE 6-WEEK SALT SOLUTION WORKOUT PLAN

WEEK	DAY 1	DAY 2	DAY 3	DAY 4	DAY 5	DAY 6	DAY 7
1	Interval Walk (35 minutes)	Steady-State Walk (40 minutes)	Interval Walk (35 minutes)	Power Walk (30 minutes)	Interval Walk (35 minutes)	Recuperative Walk (50 minutes)	Rest
	OFF	Strength training (2 sets, 15 reps, 45–60 seconds rest)	OFF	OFF	Strength training (2 sets, 15 reps, 45–60 seconds rest)	OFF	
2	Interval Walk (35 minutes)	Steady-State Walk (40 minutes)	Interval Walk (35 minutes)	Power Walk (30 minutes)	Interval Walk (35 minutes)	Recuperative Walk (1 hour)	Rest
	OFF	Strength training (2 sets, 12 reps, 30–45 seconds rest)	OFF	OFF	Strength training (2 sets, 12 reps, 30–45 seconds rest)	OFF	
3	Interval Walk (40 minutes)	Steady-State Walk (55 minutes)	Interval Walk (40 minutes)	Power Walk (40 minutes)	Interval Walk (40 minutes)	Recuperative Walk (1 hour 10 minutes)	Rest
	Strength training (2 sets, 15 reps, 45–60 seconds rest)	OFF	Strength training (2 sets, 12 reps, 30–45 seconds rest)	OFF	Strength training (2 sets, 10 reps, 15–30 seconds rest)	OFF	

WEEK	DAY 1	DAY 2	DAY 3	DAY 4	DAY 5	DAY 6	DAY 7
4	Interval Walk (40 minutes)	Steady-State Walk (55 minutes)	Interval Walk (40 minutes)	Power Walk (40 minutes)	Interval Walk (40 minutes)	Recupera-tive Walk (1 hour 20 minutes)	Rest
	Strength training (2 sets, 15 reps, 45–60 seconds rest)	OFF	Strength training (2 sets, 12 reps, 30–45 seconds rest)	OFF	Strength training (2 sets, 10 reps, 15–30 seconds rest)	OFF	
5	Interval Walk (45 minutes)	Steady-State Walk (1 hour 10 minutes)	Interval Walk (45 minutes)	Power Walk (50 minutes)	Interval Walk (45 minutes)	Recupera-tive Walk (1 hour 30 minutes)	Rest
	Strength training (3 sets, 15 reps, 45–60 seconds rest)	OFF	Strength training (3 sets, 12 reps, 30–45 seconds rest)	OFF	Strength training (3 sets, 10 reps, 15–30 seconds rest)	OFF	
6	Interval Walk (45 minutes)	Steady-State Walk (1 hour 10 minutes)	Interval Walk (45 minutes)	Power Walk (50 minutes)	Interval Walk (45 minutes)	Recupera-tive Walk (1 hour 40 minutes)	Rest
	Strength training (3 sets, 15 reps, 45–60 seconds rest)	OFF	Strength training (3 sets, 12 reps, 30–45 seconds rest)	OFF	Strength training (3 sets, 10 reps, 15–30 seconds rest)	OFF	

Salt Solution Success Story

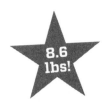

8.6 lbs!

Gretchen Tonno

Age: 49

Pounds Lost: 8.6

Inches Lost: 4½ overall

GRETCHEN, A 49-YEAR-OLD INSURANCE MARKETING MANAGER, was an athletic, fit teenager but started gaining weight in college. She gained even more in her first years of marriage; and with her two pregnancies, she found herself very unhappy with her weight in her 40s. "I've been so frustrated—nothing seemed to work." Until the Salt Solution, that is. On this program, Gretchen lost an amazing 6.2 percent body fat in only 6 weeks!

Gretchen appreciated the 2-Week Cleanse period because it made things simple for her. "Having a set meal plan made for the first 2 weeks definitely made it easy. Before, every time I tried to diet, I just found I would slack off because I couldn't find the time to plan. The Cleanse got me started on the right track."

Gretchen was surprised at how much salt she had been eating. She had never added salt to her food, so she assumed her sodium intake was under control. After peering at labels and investigating the food she ate, she realized she was wrong. "Now, I'm more cautious about what I buy. I never knew how much salt was in the foods I ate!" She was also pleasantly surprised that her energy levels skyrocketed on the Salt Solution, giving her the motivation and the get-up-and-go to exercise.

After learning (and losing weight on) the Salt Solution way of eating, Gretchen wants to change her entire family's way of eating. "The plan showed me that the portions we ate were out of control. I've been reducing serving sizes and giving my family better snacks like fruit, frozen yogurt, and veggies." Gretchen and her husband, Michael, found that they love following the Salt Solution together. "Mike and I are really helping each other stay strong so we keep losing weight."

SALT SOLUTION MAKEOVER

Gretchen's "**Before**" Diet

- **BREAKFAST:** Coffee with half-and-half, 1½ cups corn flakes, 1% milk, ½ banana
- **LUNCH:** 2 slices of pizza, salad with dressing
- **SNACK:** Apple
- **DINNER:** 2 marinated chicken breasts, green beans, dinner rolls
- **SNACK:** 6 oz ice cream

"**Before**" Nutrition

- **Calories:** 2,714
- **Sodium:** 4,065 mg
- **Saturated Fat:** 43 g
- **Fiber:** 20 g

Gretchen's "**After**" Diet

- **BREAKFAST:** Almond, Blueberry, and Banana Smoothie
- **SNACK:** Apple
- **LUNCH:** Spinach salad with mango, walnuts, and chicken breast topped with lemon juice and olive oil
- **DINNER:** Steamed Salmon
- **SNACK:** Cranberries-on-a-Banana

"**After**" Nutrition

- **Calories:** 1,403
- **Sodium:** 669 mg
- **Saturated Fat:** 8 g
- **Fiber:** 26 g

Salt Solution Improvements: With the Salt Solution, Gretchen slashed her calories almost in half (from 2,714 to 1,403 calories per day) and cut her sodium intake by *600 percent* (from 4,065 mg to 669 mg)! Gretchen lost almost 9 pounds and 4½"after 6 weeks of the Salt Solution. She also shifted her blood pressure into the healthy range, with a reading of 140/90 mmHg at the beginning of the program and 120/80 mmHg at the end of 6 weeks.

10

LIVING the Salt SOLUTION WAY

Congratulations! You've finished all 6 weeks of the Salt Solution Diet! At this point, you should be feeling leaner, less bloated, and full of energy. Maybe you've noticed a difference on the scale (or in the waistband of your pants!). Whatever effects you're noticing, you should be proud of yourself for sticking with the program.

But the Salt Solution isn't only a 6-week program. It's a plan you can follow until you reach your final weight-loss goals, and for the rest of your life. After all, you've already gone through the 2-Week Salt Solution Cleanse and the 4-Week Shake the Salt Meal Plan, and your taste buds are now accustomed to low-salt ingredients, fresh fruits and veggies, lean protein, and filling fiber. I bet you're enjoying looking leaner and feeling energized. Why turn back now? Here are a few guidelines to keep you following the Salt Solution.

Keep Salt Low: You've left the processed, packaged, high-salt foods behind you. Over the past 6 weeks, your taste buds have reset to adapt to the lower levels of salt in the Salt Solution. Along the way, you've eaten delicious, healthy, filling foods packed with vitamins and minerals. But just as your taste buds adapted to the lower salt levels of the Salt Solution, they can quickly become reaccustomed to that unhealthy, high-sodium stuff. So stick with the principles you've learned from the Salt Solution and keep salt low.

Eat Consistently: Yes, it seems contradictory, but as you now know, skipping meals won't help you lose weight. Going too many hours between meals sends your blood sugar plummeting, which can spike hunger and cause overeating. When you eat consistent meals, your energy levels stay up, your metabolism keeps humming, and your blood sugar and hunger levels are controlled. With your hunger in check, you'll be less tempted by unhealthy, high-salt, fattening snacks.

Eat Small Meals: The Salt Solution plan is designed for you to have a small meal every 4 to 5 hours, and you should stick with that schedule after the 6 weeks are over. Eating smaller meals more frequently throughout the day will keep your hunger in check. Once you reach your final weight-loss goal, add 200 calories to one of your meals (or 100 calories to two meals). After a week, weigh yourself at your usual time on your usual scale. If you have lost any weight, add another 200 calories; if you have gained any weight, drop your intake by 100 calories. Repeat until your weight has stabilized to reach the number of calories you need each day for weight maintenance.

Read Labels: You're going to need to be a sodium sleuth. Whenever you pick up a new packaged food, check the salt level. You want to stick with products with no more than about 1 milligram of sodium per calorie.

Be a Product Spy: When you're at the grocery store, keep your eyes out for new low-salt products. We've listed some of our favorite low-sodium products in this book, but manufacturers are releasing new products all the time. Look for new products, check the labels, and you might just find your new favorite low-salt snack!

Don't Beat Yourself Up: We all make mistakes. It's inevitable that you'll slip up one day and have most of a bag of chips, an extra scoop of ice cream, or a few too many margaritas. These mistakes aren't important. What is important is how you handle these roadblocks. Do you accept the mistake and start right back on the plan with the next meal? Or do you call yourself a failure and throw the plan out the window? Don't beat yourself up. It's more important to stick with the Salt Solution over the long term than to be perfect for a week.

Exercise: Exercise is your secret weapon. When you add exercise to the Salt Solution plan, you'll burn more calories, lose more weight, reduce stress, and combat disease. Stick with our activity plan or figure out your own. As long as you make exercise fun, you'll keep with it. I promise you'll enjoy the results!

Keep Stress in Check: Even though it's calorie free, stress can cause you to gain weight. Anxiety can increase blood pressure and drive you to self-medicate with unhealthy, high-salt food. One secret to long-term weight loss is keeping stress under control. Figure out your nonfood stress relievers (taking a walk, chatting with a friend) and use them whenever you feel yourself getting anxious.

Watch the Scale: You should keep up the weekly weigh-ins even after you've finished the 6 weeks of the Salt Solution. They will ensure that you're staying on the right track. If you notice the number on the scale starting to creep up, take a look at what you've been eating during the past week, whether you've been exercising, and whether you've been under stress. If you find that you need a weight-loss boost, you can always restart the Salt Solution, beginning with the 2-Week Salt Solution Cleanse. The Cleanse is a good go-to plan that you can use again and again either to jump-start weight loss or to detox after a decadent vacation. But keep in mind that the Cleanse is too low in calories to follow for long-term weight loss, and it should be used no more than twice in a 4-month period.

A Final Word

THROUGH THE SALT SOLUTION, you've learned just how many foods are packed with sodium, how salt harms our health and causes us to gain weight, and how eating low salt food can be delicious and satisfying. The Salt Solution plan is based on the latest research and has been proven effective in our test panel.

Together, members of the test panel lost a collective 140 pounds and 87¾ inches overall after only 6 weeks of the Salt Solution. True, the success is up to you. "Sometimes it's not easy," admits one of our panelists, Michael Tonno. "But the results are worth it." As our panelists found, the Salt Solution recipes are easy to prepare and delicious. "The recipes are filling, and not only do they *sound* appealing, they actually *taste* good," explains Shannon Ferry.

You may even find that you're saving money by cooking food at home and purchasing fruits, vegetables, and whole grains instead of prepared, packaged, or restaurant meals.

After 6 weeks of the Salt Solution, your relationship with food will likely change—it did for many of our test panelists. "With the Salt Solution, I have become more conscious of food. I'm not mindlessly grabbing something just to eat it. I know that ultimately I can eat whatever I want, but now what I want to eat are foods that are going to make me feel good. If I eat that cheeseburger and fries, later on I am going to feel bad not just mentally but also physically. When I eat the foods and follow the recipes on this plan, my body and mind feel so good and so satisfied that I don't want 'bad' foods anymore," says Shannon. According to panelist Mark Fatzinger, "Now that the 6 weeks of the Salt Solution have officially ended, I'm not in a hurry to rush back into my old habits. I enjoy what I'm eating!"

As Shannon says, "I was ready to make a significant change in my lifestyle. I was willing to change my attitude toward food and get my life back on track. I was done feeling bad about myself and ready to face the battle of changing my poor habits." Are you ready?

If you stick with the Salt Solution Diet, I'm confident that the plan will help you lose weight, lower your blood pressure, and live a healthier life. Good luck!

Appendix
Where to Find the Miracle Minerals

THE SALT SOLUTION PROGRAM limits your sodium intake while you increase potassium, calcium, and magnesium. These three Miracle Minerals counteract the negative effects of excess sodium, and while most people's current sodium intakes far exceed recommended levels, by contrast, our intake of these important minerals is remarkably low.

Adults need between 1,000 and 1,300 milligrams of calcium per day (depending on their age), 4,700 milligrams of potassium, and between 310 and 420 milligrams of magnesium (depending on their age and gender). But if you're like most Americans, you're getting about half as much of these minerals as you should.

The following charts are based on information from the USDA's National Nutrient Database for Standard Reference, which is used in food policy, research, and nutrition monitoring. They list the foods where you can find the Miracle Minerals per standard amount, so you can be sure to get your fill! (The reference or standard amount is the amount of food customarily eaten at one time, as set by the FDA. Serving sizes listed on food labels must be close to these reference amounts.)

★ Salt Solution Stars

The Salt Solution Stars are packed with either calcium, potassium, or magnesium—and many are great sources of all three!

STAR, STANDARD AMOUNT	POTASSIUM (MG)	CALCIUM (MG)	MAGNESIUM (MG)	CALORIES
★ **Banana,** 1 medium	422	6	32	105
★ **Beet greens,** cooked, ½ cup	655	82	49	19
★ **Halibut,** cooked, 3 oz	490	51	91	119
★ **Kale,** cooked, ½ cup	148	90	12	20
★ **Milk,** fat-free, 1 cup	382	299	27	83
★ **Sardines,** Atlantic, in oil, drained, 3 oz	338	325	33	177
★ **Soybeans,** green, cooked, ½ cup	485	130	54	127
★ **Soymilk,** calcium-fortified, 1 cup	343	340	47	109
★ **Spinach,** cooked, ½ cup	419	122	78	21
★ **Sweet potato,** baked, 1 potato (146 g)	694	55	39	131
★ **White beans,** canned, ½ cup	595	96	67	153
★ **Yogurt,** fat-free, plain, 8 oz	579	454	43	127

Source: USDA

Food Sources of Potassium

In addition to the Salt Solution Stars, many other foods are rich in potassium, including fish, legumes, and many vegetables.

FOOD, REFERENCE AMOUNT	POTASSIUM (MG)	CALORIES
Sweet potato, baked, 1 potato (146 g)	694	131
Tomato paste, ¼ cup	664	54
Beet greens, cooked, ½ cup	655	19
Potato, baked, flesh, 1 potato (156 g)	610	145
White beans, canned, ½ cup	595	153
Yogurt, fat-free, plain, 8 oz	579	127
Tomato puree, ½ cup	549	48
Clams, canned, 3 oz	534	126
Yogurt, low-fat, plain, 8 oz	531	143
Prune juice, ¾ cup	530	136
Carrot juice, ¾ cup	517	71
Blackstrap molasses, 1 Tbsp	498	47
Halibut, cooked, 3 oz	490	119
Soybeans, green, cooked, ½ cup	485	127
Lima beans, cooked, ½ cup	484	104
Tuna, yellowfin, cooked, 3 oz	484	118
Winter squash, cooked, ½ cup	448	40
Soybeans, mature, cooked, ½ cup	443	149
Rockfish, Pacific, cooked, 3 oz	442	103
Cod, Pacific, cooked, 3 oz	439	89
Banana, 1 medium	422	105
Spinach, cooked, ½ cup	419	21
Tomato juice, ¾ cup	417	31
Tomato sauce, ½ cup	405	39
Peaches, dried, uncooked, ¼ cup	398	96
Prunes, stewed, ½ cup	398	133
Milk, fat-free, 1 cup	382	83
Pork chop, center loin, cooked, 3 oz	382	197
Apricots, dried, uncooked, ¼ cup	378	78
Rainbow trout, farmed, cooked, 3 oz	375	144

FOOD, REFERENCE AMOUNT	POTASSIUM (MG)	CALORIES
Pork loin, center rib (roasts), lean, roasted, 3 oz	371	190
Buttermilk, cultured, low-fat, 1 cup	370	98
Cantaloupe, 1/4 medium	368	47
Milk, 1% or 2%, 1 cup	366	102–122
Honeydew melon, 1/8 medium	365	58
Lentils, cooked, 1/2 cup	365	115
Kidney beans, cooked, 1/2 cup	358	112
Plantains, cooked, sliced, 1/2 cup	358	90
Orange juice, 3/4 cup	355	85
Split peas, cooked, 1/2 cup	355	116
Yogurt, whole milk, plain, 8 oz	352	138

Source: USDA

Food Sources of Calcium

Dairy is, of course, a major source of this important mineral, but it isn't the only source. Here we've given you two lists, one showing which dairy foods are especially rich in calcium and one showing nondairy foods rich in calcium.

DAIRY FOOD, REFERENCE AMOUNT	CALCIUM (MG)	CALORIES
Romano cheese, 1½ oz	452	165
Yogurt, fat-free (13 g protein/8 oz), plain, 8 oz	452	127
Pasteurized process Swiss cheese, 2 oz	438	190
Yogurt, low-fat (12 g protein/8 oz), plain, 8 oz	415	143
Yogurt, low-fat (10 g protein/8 oz), fruit, 8 oz	345	232
Swiss cheese, 1½ oz	336	162
Ricotta cheese, part-skim, ½ cup	335	170
Pasteurized process American cheese food, 2 oz	323	188
Provolone cheese, 1½ oz	321	150
Mozzarella cheese, part-skim, 1½ oz	311	129
Cheddar cheese, 1½ oz	307	171
Muenster cheese, 1½ oz	305	156
Milk, fat-free, 1 cup	299	83
Milk, 1%, 1 cup	290	102
Chocolate milk, 1%, 1 cup	288	158
Chocolate milk, 2%, 1 cup	285	180
Milk, 2%, 1 cup	285	122
Buttermilk, low-fat, 1 cup	284	98
Chocolate milk, 1 cup	280	208
Whole milk, 1 cup	276	146
Yogurt, whole milk (8 g protein/8 oz), plain, 8 oz	275	138
Ricotta cheese, whole milk, ½ cup	255	214
Blue cheese, 1½ oz	225	150
Mozzarella cheese, whole milk, 1½ oz	215	128
Feta cheese, 1½ oz	210	113

Source: USDA

NONDAIRY FOOD, REFERENCE AMOUNT	CALCIUM (MG)	CALORIES
Fortified ready-to-eat cereals (various), 1 oz	236–1,043	88–106
Soymilk, calcium-fortified, 1 cup	340	109
Sardines, Atlantic, in oil, drained, 3 oz	325	177
Tofu, firm, prepared with nigari, 1/2 cup	253	88
Pink salmon, canned, with bone, 3 oz	181	118
Collards, cooked from frozen, 1/2 cup	178	31
Molasses, blackstrap, 1 Tbsp	172	47
Spinach, cooked from frozen, 1/2 cup	146	30
Soybeans, green, cooked, 1/2 cup	130	127
Turnip greens, cooked from frozen, 1/2 cup	124	24
Ocean perch, Atlantic, cooked, 3 oz	116	103
Oatmeal, plain and flavored, instant, fortified, 1 packet prepared	99–110	97–157
White beans, canned, 1/2 cup	96	153
Kale, cooked, 1/2 cup	90	20
Okra, cooked from frozen, 1/2 cup	88	26
Soybeans, mature, cooked, 1/2 cup	88	149
Blue crab, canned, 3 oz	86	84
Beet greens, cooked from fresh, 1/2 cup	82	19
Pak-choi, Chinese cabbage, cooked from fresh, 1/2 cup	79	10
Clams, canned, 3 oz	78	126
Dandelion greens, cooked from fresh, 1/2 cup	74	17
Rainbow trout, farmed, cooked, 3 oz	73	144

Source: USDA

Food Sources of **Magnesium**

Nuts, beans, and grains are good sources of magnesium.

FOOD, REFERENCE AMOUNT	MAGNESIUM (MG)	CALORIES
Pumpkin and squash seed kernels, roasted, 1 oz	151	148
Brazil nuts, 1 oz	107	186
Bran ready-to-eat cereal (100%), 1 oz	103	74
Halibut, cooked, 3 oz	91	119
Quinoa, dry, ¼ cup	89	159
Spinach, canned, ½ cup	81	25
Almonds, 1 oz	78	164
Spinach, cooked from fresh, ½ cup	78	21
Buckwheat flour, ¼ cup	75	101
Cashews, dry-roasted, 1 oz	74	163
Soybeans, mature, cooked, ½ cup	74	149
Pine nuts, dried, 1 oz	71	191
Mixed nuts, oil-roasted, with peanuts, 1 oz	67	175
White beans, canned, ½ cup	67	153
Pollock, walleye, cooked, 3 oz	62	96
Black beans, cooked, ½ cup	60	114
Bulgur, dry, ¼ cup	57	120
Oat bran, raw, ¼ cup	55	58
Soybeans, green, cooked, ½ cup	54	127
Tuna, yellowfin, cooked, 3 oz	54	118
Artichokes (hearts), cooked, ½ cup	50	42
Lima beans, baby, cooked from frozen, ½ cup	50	95
Peanuts, dry-roasted, 1 oz	50	166
Beet greens, cooked, ½ cup	49	19
Navy beans, cooked, ½ cup	48	127
Okra, cooked from frozen, ½ cup	47	26
Soy beverage, 1 cup	47	127
Tofu, firm, prepared with nigari, ½ cup	47	88
Hazelnuts, 1 oz	46	178
Oat bran muffin, 1 oz	45	77
Great Northern beans, cooked, ½ cup	44	104

FOOD, REFERENCE AMOUNT	MAGNESIUM (MG)	CALORIES
Oat bran, cooked, $\frac{1}{2}$ cup	44	44
Buckwheat groats, roasted, cooked, $\frac{1}{2}$ cup	43	78
Brown rice, cooked, $\frac{1}{2}$ cup	42	108
Haddock, cooked, 3 oz	42	95

Source: USDA

Endnotes

Introduction

1. L. H. Kuller, K. L. Margolis, S. A. Gaussoin, N. R. Bryan, D. Kerwin, M. Limacher, S. Wassertheil-Smoller, J. Williamson, and J. G. Robinson, "Relationship of Hypertension, Blood Pressure, and Blood Pressure Control with White Matter Abnormalities in the Women's Health Initiative Memory Study (WHIMS)—MRI Trial," *Journal of Clinical Hypertension* 12 (2010): 203-12.

2. F. J. He and G. A. MacGregor, "Reducing Population Salt Intake Worldwide: From Evidence to Implementation," *Progress in Cardiovascular Diseases* 52, no. 5 (2010): 363-82.

3. http://americanheart.org/presenter.jhtml?identifier=3071860.

4. http://www.americanheart.org/presenter.jhtml?identifier=4708.

5. http://www.ncbi.nlm.nih.gov/pubmed/20089957.

6. http://www.iom.edu/Reports/2010/Strategies-to-Reduce-Sodium-Intake-in-the-United-States/Report-Brief-Strategies-to-Reduce-Sodium-Intake-in-the-United-States.aspx.

7. http://www.nyc.gov/html/doh/html/pr2010/pr002-10.shtml.

8. H. Karppanen, et al., "Why and How to Implement Sodium, Potassium, Calcium, and Magnesium Changes in Food Items and Diets?" *Journal of Human Hypertension* 19 (2005): S10-S19.

Chapter 1

1. Centers for Disease Control and Prevention, "Obesity and Overweight," www.cdc.gov/nchs/fastats/overwt.htm.

2. Centers for Disease Control and Prevention, "Application of Lower Sodium Intake Recommendations to Adults—United States, 1999-2006," *MMWR Weekly* 58, no. 11 (2009): 281-83.

3. www.fitness.gov/resources_factsheet.htm.

4. H. Karppanen and E. Mervaala, "Sodium Intake and Hypertension," *Progress in Cardiovascular Diseases* 49, no. 2 (2006): 59-75.

5. F. J. He and G. A. MacGregor, "Reducing Population Salt Intake Worldwide: From Evidence to Implementation," *Progress in Cardiovascular Diseases* 52, no. 5 (2010): 363-82.

6. F. J. He, N. M. Marrero, and G. A. MacGregor, "Salt Intake Is Related to Soft Drink Consumption in Children and Adolescents," *Hypertension* 51 (2008): 629-34.

7. F. J. He, N. D. Markandu, G. A. Sagnella, and G.A. MacGregor, "Effect of Salt Intake on Renal Excretion of Water in Humans," *Hypertension* 38 (2001): 317-20.

8. M. H. Fonseca-Alaniz, L. C. Brito, C. N. Borges-Silva, J. Takada, S. Andreotti, and F. B. Lima, "High Dietary Sodium Intake Increases White Adipose Tissue Mass and Plasma Leptin in Rats," *Obesity* 15, no. 9 (2007): 2200-208.

9. M. H. Fonseca-Alaniz, J. Takada, S. Andreotti, T. B. F. de Campos, A. B. Campana, C. N. Borges-Silva, and F. B. Lima, "High Sodium Intake Enhances Insulin-Stimulated Glucose Uptake in Rat Epididymal Adipose Tissue," *Obesity* 16, no. 6 (2008): 1186–92.

10. M. J. Morris, E. S. Na, and A. K. Johnson, "Salt Craving: The Psychobiology of Pathogenic Sodium Intake," *Physiology and Behavior* 94, no. 5 (2008): 709–21.

11. F. J. He and G. A. MacGregor, "A Comprehensive Review on Salt and Health and Current Experience of Worldwide Salt Reduction Programmes," *Journal of Human Hypertension* 23, no. 6 (2009): 363–84.

12. M. H. Weinberger, N. S. Fineberg, S. E. Fineberg, and M. Weinberger, "Salt Sensitivity, Pulse Pressure, and Death in Normal and Hypertensive Humans," *Hypertension* 37 (2001): 429–32.

13 G. Danaei, E. L. Ding, D. Mozaffarian, et al., "The preventable causes of death in the United States: Comparative risk assessment of dietary, lifestyle, and metabolic risk factors," *PLoS Medicine* 6(4): e1000058. doi:10.1371/journal.pmed.1000058.

14. Crystal M. Smith-Spangler, et al., "Population Strategies to Decrease Sodium Intake and the Burden of Cardiovascular Disease," *Annals of Internal Medicine* March 1, 2010, www.annals.org/content/early/2010/02/25/0003-4819-152-8-201004200-00212.full?aimhp.

Chapter 2

1. F. J. He and G. A. MacGregor, "A Comprehensive Review on Salt and Health and Current Experience of Worldwide Salt Reduction Programmes," *Journal of Human Hypertension* 23, no. 6 (2009): 363–84.

2. E. Pimenta, K. K. Gaddam, S. Oparil, I. Aban, S. Husain, L. J. Dell'Italia, and D.A. Calhoun, "Effects of Dietary Sodium Reduction on Blood Pressure in Subjects with Resistant Hypertension: Results from a Randomized Trial," *Hypertension* 54 (2009): 475–81.

3. A. V. Diez Roux, L. Chambless, S. S. Merkin, D. Arnett, M. Eigenbrodt, F. J. Nieto, M. Szklo, and P. Sorlie, "Socioeconomic Disadvantage and Change in Blood Pressure Associated with Aging," *Circulation* 106 (2002): 703–10.

4. www.ncbi.nlm.nih.gov/pubmed/15652604.

5. M. D. Muller, E. J. Ryan, D. M. Bellar, C. Kim, M. E. Williamson, E. L. Glickman, and R. P. Blankfield, "Effect of Acute Salt Ingestion upon Core Temperature in Healthy Men," *Hypertension Research* (14 April 2011).

6. F. J. He and G. A. MacGregor, "Effect of Modest Salt Reduction on Blood Pressure: A Meta-Analysis of Randomized Trials," *Journal of Human Hypertension* 16 (2002): 761–70.

7. F. J. He and G. A. MacGregor, "Importance of Salt in Determining Blood Pressure in Children," *Hypertension* 48 (2006): 861.

8. P. Strazzullo, L. D'Elia, N. B. Kandala, and F. P. Cappuccio, "Salt Intake, Stroke, and Cardiovascular Disease: Meta-Analysis of Prospective Studies," *British Medical Journal* 339 (2009): b4567.

9. www.nhlbi.nih.gov/hbp/hbp/effect/arteries.htm.

10. K. M. Dickinson, J. B. Keogh, and P. M. Clifton, "Effects of a Low-Salt Diet on Flow-Mediated Dilation in Humans," *American Journal of Clinical Nutrition* 89 (2009): 485–90.

11. www.mayoclinic.com/health/heart-disease/DS01120.

12. www.nhlbi.nih.gov/hbp/hbp/effect/heart.htm.

13. H. C. Yu, L. M. Burrell, M. J. Black, et al., "Salt Induces Myocardial and Renal Fibrosis in Normotensive and Hypertensive Rats," *Circulation* 98 (1998): 2621–28.

14. G. du Cailar, J. Ribstein, and A. Mimran, "Dietary Sodium and Target Organ Damage in Essential Hypertension," *American Journal of Hypertension* 15 (2002): 222–29.

15. R. E. Schmieder, F. H. Messerli, H. Ruddel, et al., "Sodium Intake Modulates Left Ventricular Hypertrophy in Essential Hypertension," *Journal of Hypertension Supplement* 6 (1988): S148–50.

16. P. Strazzullo, et al., "Salt Intake, Stroke, and Cardiovascular Disease: Meta-Analysis of Prospective Studies," *British Medical Journal* 339 (2009): b4567.

17. N. R. Cook, J. A. Cutler, E. Obarzanek, J. E. Buring, K. M. Rexrode, S. K. Kumanyika, L. J. Appel, and P. K. Whelton, "Long Term Effects of Dietary Sodium Reduction on Cardiovascular Disease Outcomes: Observational Follow-Up of the Trials of Hypertension Prevention (TOHP)," *British Medical Journal* 334 (2007): 885–88.

18. www.nhlbi.nih.gov/hbp/hbp/effect/kidneys.htm.

19. H. C. Yu, L. M. Burrell, M. J. Black, et al., "Salt Induces Myocardial and Renal Fibrosis in Normotensive and Hypertensive Rats," *Circulation* 98 (1998): 2621–28.

20. B. Klanke, et al., "Blood Pressure versus Direct Mineralocorticoid Effects on Kidney Inflammation and Fibrosis in DOCA-Salt Hypertension," *Nephrology Dialysis Transplantation* 23 (2008): 3456–63.

21. www.kidney.org/kidneydisease/ckd/index.cfm#facts.

22. http://kidney.niddk.nih.gov/kudiseases/pubs/kustats/index.htm.

23. www.stroke.org/site/PageServer?pagename=STROKE.

24. www.nhlbi.nih.gov/hbp/hbp/effect/brain.htm.

25. F. J. He and G. A. MacGregor, "A Comprehensive Review on Salt and Health and Current Experience of Worldwide Salt Reduction Programmes," *Journal of Human Hypertension* 23, no. 6 (2009): 363–84.

26. www.americanheart.org/downloadable/heart/1166712318459HS_StatsInsideText.pdf.

27. P. Strazzullo, et al., "Salt Intake, Stroke, and Cardiovascular Disease: Meta-Analysis of Prospective Studies," *British Medical Journal* 339 (2009): b4567.

28. www.ncbi.nlm.nih.gov/pubmed/10941432.

29. www.ncbi.nlm.nih.gov/pubmed/17975326.

30. L. H. Kuller, K. L. Margolis, S. A. Gaussoin, N. R. Bryan, D. Kerwin, M. Limacher, S. Wassertheil-Smoller, J. Williamson, and J. G. Robinson, "Relationship of Hypertension, Blood Pressure, and Blood Pressure Control with White Matter Abnormalities in the Women's Health Initiative Memory Study (WHIMS)—MRI Trial," *Journal of Clinical Hypertension* 12 (2010): 203–12.

31. www.telegraph.co.uk/news/uknews/2262760/High-blood-pressure-increases-dementia-risk-six-fold.html.

32. J. D. Spence, "Preventing Dementia by Treating Hypertension and Preventing Stroke," *Hypertension* 44 (2004): 20.

33. T. Ogihara, T. Asano, K. Ando, Y. Chiba, N. Sekine, H. Sakoda, M. Anai, Y. Onishi, M. Fujishiro, H. Ono, N. Shojima, K. Inukai, Y. Fukushima, M. Kikuchi, and T. Fujita, "Insulin Resistance with Enhanced Insulin Signaling in High-Salt Diet-Fed Rats," *Diabetes* 50 (2001): 573–83.

34. G. Hu, et al., "Urinary Sodium and Potassium Excretion and the Risk of Type 2 Diabetes: A Prospective Study in Finland," *Diabetologia* 48, no. 8 (2005): 1477–83.

35. M. H. Fonseca-Alaniz, J. Takada, S. Andreotti, T. B. F. de Campos, A. B. Campana, C. N. Borges-Silva, and F. B. Lima, "High Sodium Intake Enhances Insulin-Stimulated Glucose Uptake in Rat Epididymal Adipose Tissue," *Obesity* 16, no. 6 (2008): 1186–92.

36. www.americanheart.org/presenter.jhtml?identifier=4756.

37. I. S. Hoffmann and L. X. Cubeddu, "Increased Blood Pressure Reactivity to Dietary Salt in Patients with the Metabolic Syndrome," *Journal of Human Hypertension* 21 (2007): 438–44.

38. www.cancer.org/cancer/cancerbasics/cancer-prevalence.

39. F. J. He and G. A. MacGregor, "Reducing Population Salt Intake Worldwide: From Evidence to Implementation," *Progress in Cardiovascular Diseases* 52, no. 5 (2010): 363–82.

40. R. Takachi, M. Inoue, T. Shimazu, S. Sasazuki, J. Ishihara, N. Sawada, T. Yamaji, M. Iwasaki, H. Iso, Y. Tsubono, and S. Tsugane; Japan Public Health Center-Based Prospective Study Group, "Consumption of Sodium and Salted Foods in Relation to Cancer and Cardiovascular Disease: The Japan Public Health Center-Based Prospective Study," *American Journal of Clinical Nutrition* 91, no. 2 (2010): 456–64.

41. www.nof.org/advocacy/prevalence/.

42. R. P. Heaney, "Role of Dietary Sodium in Osteoporosis," *Journal of the American College of Nutrition* 25 (2006): 271S–276S.

43. F. J. He and G. A. MacGregor, "Reducing Population Salt Intake Worldwide: From Evidence to Implementation," *Progress in Cardiovascular Diseases* 52, no. 5 (2010): 363–82.

44. www.cornellurology.com/sexualmedicine/ed/.

Chapter 3

1. P. Asaria, D. Chisholm, C. Mathers, M. Ezzati, and R. Beaglehole, "Chronic Disease Prevention: Health Effects and Financial Costs of Strategies to Reduce Salt Intake and Control Tobacco Use," *Lancet* 370 (2007): 2044–53.

2. K. Bibbins-Domingo, G. M. Chertow, P. G. Coxson, A. Moran, J. M. Lightwood, M. J. Pletcher, and L. Goldman, "Projected Effect on Dietary Salt Reductions on Future Cardiovascular Disease," *New England Journal of Medicine* 362 (2010): 590–99.

3. L. J. Appel, T. J. Moore, E. Obarzanek, et al., "A Clinical Trial of the Effects of Dietary Patterns on Blood Pressure. DASH Collaborative Research Group," *New England Journal of Medicine* 336 (1997): 1117–24.

4. F. M. Sacks, L. P. Svetkey, W. M. Vollmer, et al., "Effects on Blood Pressure of Reduced Dietary Sodium and the Dietary Approaches to Stop Hypertension (DASH) Diet. DASH-Sodium Collaborative Research Group," *New England Journal of Medicine* 344 (2001): 3–10.

5. H. Karppanen, et al., "Why and How to Implement Sodium, Potassium, Calcium, and Magnesium Changes in Food Items and Diets?" *Journal of Human Hypertension* 19 (2005): S10–S19.

6. National Institutes of Health, Office of Dietary Supplements, "Magnesium," http://ods.od.nih.gov/factsheets/magnesium.asp.

7. Harvard School of Public Health, "Protein: Moving Closer to Center Stage," www.hsph.harvard.edu/nutritionsource/what-should-you-eat/protein-full-story/index.html#introduction.

8. MayoClinic.com, "Can One Change Improve Your Health and the World's?" www.mayoclinic.com/health/red-meat/MY00788. Accessed on 9/23/09.

9. M. B. Zemel, W. Thompson, A. Milstead, et al., "Calcium and Dairy Acceleration of Weight and Fat Loss during Energy Restriction in Obese Adults," *Obesity Research* 12, no. 4 (2004): 582–90.

10. M. B. Zemel, J. Richards, J. Russel, A. Milstead, L. Gehardt, and E. Silva, "Dairy Augmentation of Total and Central Fat Loss in Obese Subjects," *International Journal of Obesity* 29, no. 4 (2005): 341–47.

11. Dole 5 A Day Reference Center, "Phytochemicals," http://216.255.136.121/ReferenceCenter/NutritionCenter/Phytochemicals/pdf/index.jsp?topmenu=1. Accessed on 9/23/09.

12. MayoClinic.com, "Whole Grains: Hearty Options for a Healthy Diet," www.mayoclinic.com/health/whole-grains/NU00204. Accessed on 9/23/09.

13. Harvard School of Public Health, "Health Gains from Whole Grains," www.hsph.harvard.edu/nutritionsource/what-should-you-eat/health-gains-from-whole-grains/index.html. Accessed on 9/23/09.

14. S. Liu, W. C. Willett, J. E. Manson, F. B. Hu, B. Rosner, and G. Colditz, "Relation between Changes in Intakes of Dietary Fiber and Grain Products and Changes in Weight and Development of Obesity among Middle-Aged Women," *American Journal of Clinical Nutrition* 78 (2003): 920–27.

15. P. Koh-Banerjee, M. Franz, L. Sampson, S. Liu, D. R. J. Jacobs, D. Spiegelman, W. Willett, and E. Rimm, "Changes in Whole-Grain, Bran, and Cereal Fiber Consumption in Relation to 8-Y Weight Gain among Men," *American Journal of Clinical Nutrition* 80 (2004): 1237–45.

Chapter 7

1. www.iom.edu/Reports/2010/Strategies-to-Reduce-Sodium-Intake-in-the-United-States/Report-Brief-Strategies-to-Reduce-Sodium-Intake-in-the-United-States.aspx.

2. www.huffingtonpost.com/michael-f-jacobson/health-advice-why-we-emne_b_547745.html.

3. www.nyc.gov/html/doh/html/pr2010/pr002-10.shtml.

4. www.huffingtonpost.com/2010/04/26/salt-reduction-coming-for_n_552929.html.

5. www.nhlbi.nih.gov/health/public/heart/hbp/dash/how_make_dash.html.

6. www.heart.org/HEARTORG/GettingHealthy/NutritionCenter/HealthyDietGoals/Sodium-Salt-or-Sodium-Chloride_UCM_303290_Article.jsp.

7. www.nal.usda.gov/afsic/pubs/ofp/ofp.shtml.

8. www.mayoclinic.com/health/organic-food/NU00255.

9. www.amys.com/products/category_view.php?prod_category=15.

10. www.heinzketchup.com/Products.aspx.

11. www.foodnews.org/walletguide.php.

12. www.nal.usda.gov/fnic/foodcomp/search/.

Chapter 8

1. http://nutrition.mcdonalds.com/nutritionexchange/ingredientslist.pdf.

2. C. M. Johnson, S. Y. Angell, A. Lederer, et al., "Sodium Content of Lunchtime Fast Food Purchases at Major US Chains," *Archives of Internal Medicine* 170 (2010): 732–34.

3. Cornell University, "People Eat More Stale Popcorn If Served in a Big Bucket," *ScienceDaily,* November 14, 2005. Retrieved August 4, 2010, from www.sciencedaily.com/releases/2005/11/051110221344.htm.

4. www.jneb.org/article/S1499-4046%2809%2900025-6/abstract.

Chapter 9

1. Simon J. Marshall, et al., "Translating Physical Activity Recommendations into a Pedometer-Based Step Goal: 3000 Steps in 30 Minutes," *American Journal of Preventive Medicine* 36, no. 5 (May 2009): 410–15.

2. E. Puterman, et al., "The Power of Exercise: Buffering the Effect of Chronic Stress on Telomere Length," *PLoS ONE* 5, no. 5 (2010).

3. Markus Gerber, et al., "Fitness and Exercise as Correlates of Sleep Complaints: Is It All in Our Minds?" *Medicine and Science in Sports and Exercise* 42, no. 5 (May 2010): 893–901.

4. Paul S. MacLean, et al., "Regular Exercise Attenuates the Metabolic Drive to Regain Weight after Long-Term Weight Loss," *AJP Regulatory Integrative and Comparative Physiology* 297, no. 3 (2009): R793–802.

5. Jo Barton and Jules Pretty, "What Is the Best Dose of Nature and Green Exercise for Improving Mental Health? A Multi-Study Analysis," *Environmental Science and Technology* 44, no. 10 (2010): 3947–55.

6. Gary R. Hunter, et al., "Exercise Training Prevents Regain of Visceral Fat for 1-Year Following Weight Loss," *Obesity* 18, no. 4 (2010): 690–95.

Acknowledgments

A SPECIAL NOTE OF APPRECIATION goes to Kate Mueller, MPH, RD, and Juhie Bhatia. I could not have done this book without your help! Thank you to the wonderful *Salt Solution* team: Andrea Au Levitt (the best editor ever!), David Bonom (recipe developer extraordinaire), Myatt Murphy (fastest fitness writer in the East), and Marielle Messing (tireless editorial assistant and test panel coordinator). And to the dedicated Rodale Books team, including Chris Krogermeier, Sara Cox, Hope Clarke, Carol Angstadt, Chalkley Calderwood, Anne Egan, Brooke Myers, Liz Krenos, Wendy Gable, and the *Prevention* team, especially Marlea Clark.

Thanks also to all of the people who participated in the Salt Solution test panel: Diane Anderson, Denise Battista, Melanie Cardell, Gloria Creech, Dianne Daniels, Mark Fatzinger, Shannon Ferry, Laura Gutierrez, Bonita Hill, Anne Huey, Alice Mudge, Robin Scholtz, Gretchen Tonno, Mike Tonno, Beth Vorosmarti, and Kathy Walker. Deep gratitude also goes to Kelly Hartshorne and Tammy Strunk for their help with the test panel.

Finally, thanks to my agent, Janis Donnaud.

To Aaron.
Thank you for your
unconditional love and
unwavering support.
You inspire me.

Index

Underscored page references indicate boxed text and tables. **Boldface** references indicate photographs.

Pork and Beans, <u>72</u>

Pork and Sweet Potato Skillet, 146

Pork Tenderloin with Avocado Salad, 145

Portion control, in restaurants, 220

Potassium

food sources of, 43, 45, 46, 47, <u>285</u>, <u>286–87</u>

low, health risks from, 37

in Mineral Boost Juice, 64, 81

as Miracle Mineral, 16–17, 42, 43–44

recommended daily intake of, 43, 284

Potassium chloride, in sodium-free products, <u>2</u>, 188

Potatoes

Italian Baked Fries, 157

Poultry. *See also* Chicken; Turkey

low-sodium, choosing, 194–95

Power walks, 239, <u>243</u>, <u>245</u>, <u>247</u>, <u>249</u>, <u>251</u>, <u>253</u>

Prepared foods and meals

definition of, <u>8</u>

without nutrition labels, 193

salt in, 9

reducing, 211

Pretzels

Dried Fruit, Chocolate Chip, Pretzel, and Nut Mix, 168

Processed foods

affecting taste buds, 60

definition of, <u>8</u>

low-sodium choices of, 194–97, 200–203, 206–7

minimizing use of, 185

sodium in, 9

food-industry efforts to reduce, 16, 186

in supermarkets, 193

Produce. *See also* Fruits; Vegetables

low-sodium, choosing, 197, 200

in Salt Solution diet, 50–51, 85

Progress, gauges of, <u>68</u>

Protein

low-sodium, choosing, 194–96

in Salt Solution diet, 48–49, 85

Puddings

Baked Rice and Raisin Pudding, 107

Cardamom Rice Pudding, 177

Easy Chocolate Pudding with Banana, 181

Healthy Bread Pudding, 175

Pumpkin

Pumpkin-Maple Cheesecake, 172

Q

Quinoa

Lentil Quinoa Burgers, 150

Quiz, Salt-o-Meter, <u>10–12</u>

R

Race, as disease risk factor, 35

Raisins

Baked Rice and Raisin Pudding, 107

Rate of Perceived Exertion (RPE), for gauging exercise intensity, 237–38

Recipes, Salt Solution, 18. *See also specific recipes*

mixing and matching, 81

omitting salt from, 209

overview of, 93–94

Recuperative walks, 240, <u>243</u>, <u>245</u>, <u>247</u>, <u>249</u>, <u>251</u>, <u>253</u>

Red meats, 48–49

Refrigerator staples, low-sodium, 188

Relish

Pear-Apricot Relish, <u>208</u>

Renal fibrosis, 29

Reps, in strength training, 254, 256

Restaurant foods. *See also* Dining out

guidelines for eating, 217–21

sodium in, 60, <u>65</u>

efforts to reduce, 186

Rewards, 227

Rice

Baked Rice and Raisin Pudding, 107

Cardamom Rice Pudding, 177

Rice mixes, low-sodium, 200–201

Rinsing foods, for eliminating excess salt, 209

Rosemary, <u>205</u>

Rosemary Salmon, 141

RPE scale, for gauging exercise intensity, 237–38

S

Sage, <u>205</u>

Salad dressings

alternatives to, 210

Citrus Dressing, <u>208</u>

Dressing, <u>208</u>

low-sodium, 207

sodium in, 219

Salads

Couscous and Lentil Salad, 126

Curried Egg Salad over Spinach, 124

Edamame Salad, <u>71</u>

Greens and Couscous Salad, <u>72</u>

Mediterranean Chicken Salad, 86

Middle Eastern Chopped Salad, 128

Nutty Fruit Salad, 127

Pork Tenderloin with Avocado Salad, 145

Roast Turkey, Orange, and Cashew Salad, 122

low-sodium, 197, 200
Minestrone Soup, 130
in Salt Solution diet, 50–51, 85
Spinach Hummus with Vegetable Dippers,
162
Vegetable Penne, 148
Vitamin D, for calcium absorption, 44, 50
Vorosmarti, Beth, 57, 212–13

W

Walking. *See also* Walking program
for burning extra calories, 5
Walking program
goals of, 234
when to use, 235, 236
determining exertion level of, 237
outdoor cautions about, 241
routines in, 238–40
week 1, 242–43
week 2, 244–45
week 3, 246–47
week 4, 248–49
week 5, 250–51
week 6, 252–53
Watermelon
Spice-Rubbed Chicken with Watermelon
Salad, 134
Water retention
from excess sodium, 3, 8, 26
from salt sensitivity, 13

Weigh-ins, 68, 280–81, 282
Weight gain
Miracle Minerals preventing, 45
from stress, 281
Weight loss
calcium aiding, 49–50
from 4-Week Shake the Salt Meal Plan, 79 (*see
also* Success stories)
keys to, 1
from salt restriction, 15, 41
stress management and, 281–82
from 2-Week Salt Solution Cleanse, 59, 61, 62
(*see also* Success stories)
whole grains and, 52
Whole grains. *See* Grains, whole
Wrap
Tofu-Spinach Wrap, 119

Y

Yogurt
Breakfast Berry "Sundaes," 108
Greek Yogurt with Walnuts and Honey, 109
Miracle Minerals in, 47
Orange-Yogurt Pops, 73
Yogurt Parfait with Berries, 70

Z

Zucchini
Zucchini Chips, 155

Conversion Chart

These equivalents have been slightly rounded to make measuring easier.

VOLUME MEASUREMENTS			WEIGHT MEASUREMENTS		LENGTH MEASUREMENTS	
U.S.	**IMPERIAL**	**METRIC**	**U.S.**	**METRIC**	**U.S.**	**METRIC**
¼ tsp	–	1 ml	1 oz	30 g	¼"	0.6 cm
½ tsp	–	2 ml	2 oz	60 g	½"	1.25 cm
1 tsp	–	5 ml	4 oz (¼ lb)	115 g	1"	2.5 cm
1 Tbsp	–	15 ml	5 oz (⅓ lb)	145 g	2"	5 cm
2 Tbsp (1 oz)	1 fl oz	30 ml	6 oz	170 g	4"	11 cm
¼ cup (2 oz)	2 fl oz	60 ml	7 oz	200 g	6"	15 cm
⅓ cup (3 oz)	3 fl oz	80 ml	8 oz (½ lb)	230 g	8"	20 cm
½ cup (4 oz)	4 fl oz	120 ml	10 oz	285 g	10"	25 cm
⅔ cup (5 oz)	5 fl oz	160 ml	12 oz (¾ lb)	340 g	12" (1')	30 cm
¾ cup (6 oz)	6 fl oz	180 ml	14 oz	400 g		
1 cup (8 oz)	8 fl oz	240 ml	16 oz (1 lb)	455 g		
			2.2 lb	1 kg		

PAN SIZES		TEMPERATURES		
U. S.	**METRIC**	**FAHRENHEIT**	**CENTIGRADE**	**GAS**
8" cake pan	20 X 4 cm sandwich or cake tin	140°	60°	–
9" cake pan	23 X 3.5 cm sandwich or cake tin	160°	70°	–
11" X 7" baking pan	28 X 18 cm baking tin	180°	80°	–
13" X 9" baking pan	32.5 X 23 cm baking tin	225°	105°	¼
15" X 10" baking pan	38 X 25.5 cm baking tin	250°	120°	½
	(Swiss roll tin)	275°	135°	1
1½ qt baking dish	1.5 liter baking dish	300°	150°	2
2 qt baking dish	2 liter baking dish	325°	160°	3
2 qt rectangular	30 X 19 cm baking dish	350°	180°	4
baking dish		375°	190°	5
9" pie plate	22 X 4 or 23 X 4 cm pie plate	400°	200°	6
7" or 8" springform	18 or 20 cm springform or	425°	220°	7
pan	loose-bottom cake tin	450°	230°	8
9" X 5" loaf pan	23 X 13 cm or 2 lb narrow	475°	245°	9
	loaf tin or pâté tin	500°	260°	–